Eat for Your Brain

Sue Cook BSc (Hons) Lic LCCH

SUE COOK

Copyright © 2016 Sue Cook

All rights reserved.

ISBN: 1532750943
ISBN-13: 9781532750946

DEDICATION

To all those people wanting to improve their health through food and find the answers you seek.

SUE COOK

CONTENTS

	Acknowledgments	i
1	introduction	1
2	Section 1: Look up your symptoms	17
3	Section 2 The foods described	31

	aloe vera	31
	amino acids	34
	astaxanthin	34
	barleygrass	35
	bee pollen	36
	blueberries and cranberries	37
	broccoli	38
	Brussels sprouts	38
	cabbage	38
	cacao	38
	cauliflower	39
	chaga fungus	39
	chia seeds	40
	coconut	40
	collards	42
	cordyceps	42
	cracked chlorella	42
	goji berries	46
	Himalayan Pink Salt	48
	kale	48
	kelp	49
	L-Carnitine	51
	Leafy greens	51
	lemon and citrus	51

	maca	52
	matcha	52
	presprouted barley	53
	probiotics	53
	raw sprouted seeds	56
	red algae	57
	shiitake mushrooms	57
	spinach	57
	spirulina	57
	Swiss chard	58
	walnuts	59
	watercress	60
	wheatgrass	60
4	references	63
	resources	125
	about the author	126

ACKNOWLEDGMENTS

I acknowledge my mum for being such an awesome role model.

INTRODUCTION

Eat for your brain?
I work mostly with people with learning issues, and so I am always looking for ways of improving/increasing their physical and mental development/status. So that was where I started with this book. But as you know, we aren't just a brain, we are connected to our body. Gut health is such a big issue it has been called the second brain. So even though the title is EAT FOR YOUR BRAIN, by eating for your brain you are also going to be eating for your body too. I hope you don't mind the liberty taken with the title. I thought it was catchy.

This is the book I wanted to read on super foods but couldn't find….
I'm a cynic. I want definite information. Not 'maybes'. I want real solid facts. I'm an enthusiastic researcher too. I'm also limited by the things that restrict us: time; interpretation; intelligence. So this is my shot at understanding what is worth eating and what is worth ignoring (and I may follow up with volume 2 on other super foods later).
The 'maybe's in research seem to come from when things have been tested on animals and not so well in

people. Bioavailability is a fundamental part of this. The food you are eating has to be in a form the body can use AND your body has to be able to extract the nutrients by having sufficient enzymes, stomach acid and so on. These diminish as we age and so foods are less bioavailable to us....
So the job of a good meal is to: provide maximum nutrients; AND ENABLE digestion and absorption by the body. Or it's pointless. For this to happen it often means eating certain things together.....

This book is not about meat and potatoes, that is in my other nutrition book. It's several years since we wrote Nutrition for Special Needs, and so in that time we have learnt more things and had more experiences, and the world has changed.

My motivation for sharing information on health is this: At age 19 I had what my GP said was the worst case of glandular fever on record. And it nearly killed me in that I started choking one night and saw my life flash before me. I didn't breathe for ages (maybe at least a minute or more and enough time for my mum and my sister to rush into the kitchen to look for a knife to give me a tracheotomy) and eventually I coughed. And it changed my life. My lower jaw was dislocated forward to due to the swollen glands in my neck and I couldn't eat and taking a sip of water with aspirin in it would take me ten minutes to pluck up the courage to swallow because my throat was ulcerated and raw: completely.
I was weak by the time I had choked, several weeks into the illness, and I had no energy at all. After I breathed, I was in shock. How could something so simple as a virus

nearly kill off a strong healthy 19 year old? We had been told nothing could be done, it was a virus. So began my quest, upon my recovery, to find ways of acquiring great health and resistance. This illness had scared me and it changed my life totally. Since then, (and that was 31 years ago) I have been learning and researching. I've written other books on what I have found, in the areas of learning issues and nutrition for special needs, but this is the first book for the general public. So for the last 31 years my health has been a colossal priority in my life. I even trained as a health scientist, being taught my medical doctors. I've had a private health care practice for 20 years.

A lot of people find research papers boring and frightening so the majority are in the references section. Just a few are here with relevant quotes.

This book is about foods not supplements (in the main), though some of these foods come in pill or powder form they are still foods...Problems with supplements can be toxicity: there is research that discusses toxicity of selenium supplementation. It seems from study and experience that eating foods is better than taking supplements, because isolating a substance to focus on one aspect of its action can create an imbalance. So if we eat a range of foods that have several (or many) important ingredients, then we are bypassing the risk of inadvertently poisoning ourselves. Just look at the list of nutrients that many of these foods have and you will see what I mean. And compare that with taking a sudden massive amount of one nutrient... *Science of The Total Environment Volume 400, Issues 1–3, 1 August 2008, Pages 115–141 Selenium in food and the human body: A review Miguel Navarro-Alarcon, , Carmen Cabrera-Vique*
British Journal of Nutrition
This paper showed benefit to cancer patients by supplementation of essential fats, and is a systematic review of literature. *British Journal of Nutrition / Volume 97 / Issue 05 / May 2007, pp 823-831Copyright © The Authors 2007 DOI: http://dx.doi.org/*

10.1017/S000711450765795X (About DOI), Published online: 05 April 2007.

These last two papers show very different standpoints on supplementation. When faced with what might seem like contradictory information in scientific papers (because it is possible to search for pro and cons of almost everything), several things may be considered. We are all individuals, all have unique responses to our environments. We must eat. So somewhere on this journey we are going to find things that suit us and things that don't. Use the information as a tool rather than a directive. Do what works for you. In my case, a mixture of normal food, super foods and occasional supplements enables me to feel great.

The aim of this book is to help you find your way to stay healthy, despite conflicting information, if it works for you, it works.

What this is and what this isn't:

Everything in this book comes from research, listed at the end (except in the introduction). The aim of Section 1 and Section 2 in this book is to find information quickly, such as 'what can I eat to heal my — — symptoms?'
Look up the food in section 2.
Look up the research if you so choose, in the references at the back. The research is not cluttering the bits you want to access quickly (sections 1 and 2). If I was going to reference each piece of information, it would make it harder to read so I have put it separately. I do not go into analysis here, you can do that from the research I list.

- I'm a health scientist not a nutritionist.
- I have 20 years in practice helping patients. This book is not designed to be definitive but to be useful and practical.

- What is a superfood?
these are super healthy things to eat. I'd not heard of most of them when I was a kid.
- Why do we need a book on it?
When I was researching this I couldn't find the right information in any books, so I thought I had to create the book I wanted to read.
- Who needs it?

Those concerned with their health, wanting to stay young, anti ageing, prevention, and those interested in their nutrition.
* What can you achieve?

Better health, recovery, delayed ageing, rejuvenation of the body.
* What do super foods do that normal foods can't?

Superfoods have more nutrients in them so they can achieve more good things for the body than empty calories can or 'inferior' foods. They can actively help you heal and reverse health conditions by giving your body what it needs.
* These are not supplements, they are foods that heal (in the main).

Sugar Addiction

Last summer I discovered a way to break the sugar addiction that I had. It took ten days and it was life changing. My blood sugar was stable and my mood was even, and I lost weight.

I have found that I didn't need or miss sugar and that I wasn't dependent on it. I had kept it at bay for years, but I hadn't beaten it. This ten day 'cleanse' changed all that.

That was my first total immersion in super foods and I loved it. I could see the scope and wanted to know everything I could, and how to apply this to my patients. So I have been using super foods and seeing what is possible.

For more information on this specific cleanse, go to www.mypuriumgift.com and type in brainbuzzz in the gift card code (note the 3 Z) when prompted. Look for the ten day cleanse.

Many chronic diseases boil down to:
* malnutrition
* poor digestion

Free radicals and disease: Oxford Journals Medicine & Health British Medical Bulletin Volume 49, Issue 3Pp. 679-699.
Prospects for the prevention of free radical disease, regarding cancer and cardiovascular disease
Toxic Proteins in Neurodegenerative Disease
J. Paul Taylor1,*, John Hardy2, Kenneth H. Fischbeck1
Science 14 Jun 2002: Vol. 296, Issue 5575, pp. 1991-1995 DOI: 10.1126/science.1067122

'Antioxidants are needed to prevent the formation and oppose the actions of reactive oxygen and nitrogen species, which are generated in vivo and cause damage to DNA, lipids, proteins, and other biomolecules. Endogenous antioxidant defenses (superoxide dismutases, H2O2-removing enzymes, metal binding proteins) are inadequate to prevent damage completely, so diet derived antioxidants are important in maintaining health.'
Antioxidants in Human Health and Disease Annual Review of Nutrition Vol. 16: 33-50 (Volume publication date July 1996) DOI: 10.1146/annurev.nu.16.070196.000341 Barry Halliwell Pharmacology Group, King's College, University of London, Manresa Road, London SW3 6LX, United Kingdom
The American Journal of Clinical Nutrition by The American Society for Clinical Nutrition, Inc Synergism of nutrition, infection, and immunity: an overview. N S Scrimshaw and J P SanGiovanni
'Infection and malnutrition have always been intricately linked. Malnutrition is the primary cause of immunodeficiency worldwide... Five infectious diseases account for more than one-half of all deaths in children aged <5 years, most of whom are undernourished' Oxford Journals Medicine & Health Clinical Infectious Diseases Volume 46, Issue 10Pp. 1582-1588. The Interaction between Nutrition and Infection Peter Katona1 and Judit Katona-Apte2,a The David Geffen School of Medicine at the University of California at Los Angeles, Los Angeles
United Nations World Food Program, Rome, Italy

Dr. Peter Katona, The David Geffen School of Medicine at UCLA, 100 UCLA Medical Plaza, Ste. 310, Los Angeles, CA 90024 (pkatona@ucla.edu).
'Diet is estimated to contribute to about one-third of preventable cancers — about the same amount as smoking.' What is possible with the right foods is good health. Nature Reviews Cancer 2, 694-704 (September 2002) I doi:10.1038/nrc886 Are vitamin and mineral deficiencies a major cancer risk? Bruce N. Ames1 & Patricia Wakimoto1

Super foods address malnutrition and digestion

Superfoods are strongly alkali (meat, dairy and grains are acidifying to the body).

Acid foods maintain alkalinity in the body by pulling minerals from the bones and other tissues to buffer the acidity. In other words eating the wrong foods depletes the body of minerals.

Enzymes will be moved from other areas of the body (there are several different types that do different things in the body) to the gut to break down food when there is a deficiency, and the person will age rapidly, and get degenerative conditions.

Decreased enzymes have been shown to be present in allergies, skin disease, cancer and diabetes.

* Why are they good for the brain?

The brain depends on certain things to function optimally. Good fats, and so on, and without this, thinking can be slow, damaged, not happening, foggy, reactions can be slow, memory impaired and so on. Who wants that? Not me.

The Compound Effect

* The compound effect! The effect of healthy living every day has a big impact over time. The compound effect of heavy drinking, drug taking, poor diet builds up over time. Which will you choose?

Look at this way, if you are born very strong and you take it for granted and don't look after your health, at some point you will be overtaken in health by the people born less strong who do healthy things every day and build on and maintain a healthy mind and body right into old age.

Would you rather have a million pounds now or a penny doubled every day for 31 days (a month)? After a month the £1 Million is still a million but the penny is worth £10 million. The same principle applies for your health, good habits pay dividends in the long run and the short.

http://www.thecompoundeffect.com/

●What must be working for health?:

Digestion

(because we eat the super foods and we want to absorb the nutrition)

Digestion relies on enzymes and probiotic bacteria. Deficiency of these results in:
constipation
arthritis
gastritis
allergies
candida
obesity
acne
BO
Overacidity results in:
hernia
See the importance of good gut health!

Let's look at one ingredient and its impact: Chlorophyll
<u>In the Mouth:</u>
Chlorophyll can immediately help:
bleeding gums
canker sores
gingivitis
sore throats
anticancer
in the oesophagus
heartburn
reflux
alkali effect of chlorophyll

<u>in the stomach</u>
chlorophyll eliminates helico bacter pylori (stomach ulcers and stomach cancer)

<u>in the small intestine and liver</u>
once absorbed chlorophyll promotes the liver's cancer neutralising enzymes
and inhibits dioxin (pollutants) absorption

<u>in the colon</u>
increased elimination of toxins and cancer causing agents, increase motility, internal deodoriser.
Details here are from The Superfoods Bible by David Sandoval, Panacea Publishing, www.PanaceaPublishingInc.com. 2015.

Deficiency Symptoms
magnesium (I mention this because it is s prevalent these days)
how to get magnesium from super foods: chlorella, cacao
Combinations
how to put together the super foods: sweet/savoury
how to gauge what to do as you go

how to tell what's going on according to your symptoms (migraines on cracked chlorella indicating magnesium deficiency), thyroid, stress...

Nutritional Kryptonite
Various foods seem to be kryptonite to some people, but I do not address those issues here. See my other book: Nutrition for Special Needs. Here is a little taster here for you of symptoms a sensitive person can get from eating the wrong things:
Gluten
- A protein (not a carb) that can be very hard to digest.

●Symptoms of gluten intolerance:
- digestive issues
- mood swings
- brain fog
- balance issues
- tingling
- headaches
- fatigue
- autoimmune skin conditions like eczema or psoriasis (improved by oxygenating foods)
- fibromyalgia
- hormonal imbalance
- keratosis pilaris: bumps and hard skin on thighs, arms, cheeks
- joint pain
- swelling
- dental issues from results of inflammation on the body

- Sugar
- makes you fat and acidifies the body

Heavy metals

- Whats the big deal with heavy metals? Smoking, eating fish, dental amalgams, lead in petrol, arsenic in water, have all contributed to contaminating us with these metals.
- Imagine a farm that grows vegetables, and a terrace of houses. The houses are supposed to be for the trained farmers who know how to plant, harvest, nurture the crops. But the workers can't live there and do their job because the house has been taken over by a violent gang. So the crops don't get planted, tended to or harvested and so the people who need the crops die of starvation. That is the effect of heavy metals on the body. The chlorella (or other food that gets rid of heavy metals) goes into the houses and escorts the violent gang out of the farm so that the workers can return.

Br Med Bull (2003) 68 (1): 167-182. doi: 10.1093/bmb/ldg032
This article appears in: Impact of environmental pollution on health: Balancing risk heavy metals accumulate and thereby disrupt function in vital organs and glands such as the heart, brain, kidneys, bone, liver, etc.

'*They displace the vital nutritional minerals from their original place, thereby, hindering their biological function. There are many ways by which these toxins can be introduced into the body such as consumption of foods, beverages, skin exposure, and the inhaled air*'.
Indian J Pharmacol. 2011 May-Jun; 43(3): 246–253. doi: 10.4103/0253-7613.81505 PMCID: PMC3113373 Heavy metals and living systems: An overview Reena Singh, Neetu Gautam, Anurag Mishra, and Rajiv GuptaSection 1

'Heavy metals stop enzymes from working by affecting the tertiary structures by catalysing protein destroying reactions or interfering with sulphur-sulphur cross bridges' effectively rendering the enzyme useless. https://www.google.co.uk/url?sa=t&rct=j&q=&esrc=s&source=web&cd=1&cad=rja&uact=8&ved=0ahUKEwjwmoXK9fnLAhVELhoKHfSrCCUQFggcMAA&url=http%3A%2F%2Fwww.sd67.bc.ca%2Fschools%2Fsalc%2Fbiology%252012%2Fmodule%2520b%2520-%2520cell%2520processes%2520and%2520applications%2Funit%25208%2520-%2520enzymes%2Fheavymetal.pdf&usg=AFQjCNFvaRz-EaDR8iU3jH1RRz7vYdFUNQ&sig2=YNhIbdCnt4Bq-VZpOoA2Nw

In Conclusion to prevent malnutrition and poor digestion we need:
- enzymes
- bioavailable nutrients
- high quality nutrients
- nutrients that are safe and in the right balance and combination

Looking at the evidence, some foods described below are safe all the time, and some need to be consumed with other foods:
- For example, with kombucha liver toxicity has been described when used for several months daily. There is also overwhelming evidence to support the use of kombucha. These two opposite findings are from peer reviewed gold standard trials. So, it would seem sensible, if one is to consume this, to not have it daily, and to take breaks of several weeks every few months. Furthermore, in the papers I have reviewed, it does not state the original nutritional status of the individuals and whether they are taking an across the board super foods approach to their nutrition. If they were, and they were consuming liver supporting foods, then the toxicity issue may never occur.

This further reinforces the need to improve nutrition to a higher standard in those individuals who benefit from kombucha and not to rely on a single substance to heal us. I'm recommending a combination of these.

Other Combinations:
- Matcha must be consumed with chlorella to overcome the lead potential
- Chlorella must be consumed with enzymes

- Raw cabbage, broccoli and cauliflower can suppress the thyroid and worsen acne so take with himalayan pink salt
- 1.1mg of Kelp maximum as it can create hyperthyroidism and it is not a safe weight loss food as it can create a hyper-thyroid state
- Goji berry issues: migraines
- Maca is not recommended in hormonal cancers
- Walnuts and peanuts contain high levels of L-Arginine by reducing lysine levels which can trigger herpes virus in those who have it.
- Tuna: eat with kelp or cracked chlorella incase of heavy metal content.

- I'm not into recipes. I hate cooking, but I am passionate about health. What I like about super foods is that I can bung them in the Nutri Ninja and have a meal prepared ready to drink in two minutes. You can get recipes from other authors.

Let me introduce the super foods with which you may be unfamiliar.

Matcha comes in a powder. It is a tea. It is green. I use one teaspoon.
Maca comes in a power. It is a tuberous root like a potato. It is yellow. I use one teaspoon.
chlorella comes in powder and tablet form. It is a seaweed. it is green. I take up to 20 tablets three times a day.
spirulina comes in powder and tablet form. It is a seaweed. It is green. I take 5 tablets three times a day.
wheatgrass comes powdered and juiced. It is the young shoots of wheat but contains no gluten. It is green. I take a teaspoon.
barleygrass comes powdered and juiced. It is the young shoots of barley but contains no gluten.It is green. I take a teaspoon but you can take up to three tablespoons.
Chaga comes in chunks, powdered and in a tea. It is a mushroom. It is brown. There are videos on YouTube where you can see it being prepared.
Astaxanthin comes in capsules and powder. It is the red/pink colour in seafood. It is pink/red. One capsule, but in the case of athletes or those with joint problems, take two. Eat with food.

kelp comes in powder, tablets, and capsules. It is seaweed. It is green. 600-1200mg per meal.
Pre-sprouted barley comes in freshly sprouted seed form, and powder. It is sprouted seeds. It is white and yellow. There are some good videos on YouTube about sprouting.

All of these are savoury except for maca which can be added to fruit smoothies. All of these can be added to smoothies except chaga which you can take as a tea. When I buy a bag of kale, I put it in the freezer, and when it is frozen, I break it up and then it takes up less space and I can grab a handful for the blender.

Quantities
When you buy these products, the dosage is listed on the package. In the case of fresh foods, eat what feels right.
Most of these can be bought from the whole food shop, the supermarket or online. I get most of mine from Purium at www.mypuriumgiftcard.com as described above.

How nutrition fits in to exercise
There is a lot of research on the importance of the right nutrition for athletes, as they are using their body for hard training and recovery is key to maintaining high performance. Non athletes (like me) will still be impacted by what we eat in relation to our exercise and recovery. But on a more subtle scale. I have selected a few research paper references and quotes to show you how it is a known and accepted fact that food and exercise need to be in harmony for maximum health.
Elite athlete immunology: importance of nutrition.
(PMID:10893024)
Abstract
Gleeson M , Bishop NC
School of Sport and Exercise Sciences, University of Edgbaston, Birmingham, England. m.gleeson@bham.ac.uk
International Journal of Sports Medicine [2000, 21 Suppl 1:S44-50]
'By adopting sound nutritional practice, reducing other life stresses, maintaining good hygiene, obtaining adequate rest and spacing prolonged training sessions and competition as far apart

as possible, athletes can reduce their risk of infection.mental/brain health is partly affected by gut health'
Importance of exercise and nutrition in the prevention of illness and the enchancement of health
Akande, A; C de W van Wyk; Osagie, J E. Education120.4 (Summer 2000): 758-772.

We can't separate ourselves into bits, so eating for your brain is also eating for your gut and your total welfare.
Current Sports Medicine Reports:
July/August 2008 - Volume 7 - Issue 4 - pp 193-201
doi: 10.1249/JSR.0b013e31817fc0fd
Recovery Nutrition: Timing and Composition after Endurance Exercise
Millard-Stafford, Melinda; Childers, W. Lee; Conger, Scott A.; Kampfer, Angela J.; Rahnert, Jill A.
Nutrition for post-exercise recovery.
(PMID:9127682)

Burke LM
Australian Institute of Sport, ACT, Australia.
Australian Journal of Science and Medicine in Sport [1997, 29(1): 3-10]

Protein ingestion before sleep improves postexercise overnight recovery.
(PMID:22330017)
Res PT , Groen B , Pennings B , Beelen M , Wallis GA , Gijsen AP , Senden JM , VAN Loon LJ
Department of Human Movement Sciences, NUTRIM School for Nutrition, Toxicology and Metabolism, Maastricht University Medical Centre+, Maastricht, The Netherlands.
Medicine and Science in Sports and Exercise [2012, 44(8): 1560-1569]
'Training relies heavily on the athlete's tolerance to repetitive strain. Today's ultra-endurance athlete must also follow appropriate nutritional practices in order to recover and prepare for daily training and remain injury free and healthy. Rehydration after exercise, together with the timing and method of increased food intake to cope with heavy training, are essential for optimal performance. Furthermore, the treatment of soft tissue after

training or racing is necessary to control inflammation.' Current Sports Medicine Reports May 2005, Volume 4, Issue 3, pp 165-170
First online: 24 March 2014 Training principles and issues for ultra-endurance athletes Calvin Zaryski, David J. Smith

'Appropriate nutrition is an essential prerequisite for effective improvement of athletic performance, conditioning, recovery from fatigue after exercise, and avoidance of injury.' Exercise and functional foods Wataru AoiEmail author, Yuji Naito and Toshikazu Yoshikawa
Nutrition Journal20065:15 DOI: 10.1186/1475-2891-5-15© Aoi et al. 2006 Published: 05 June 2006

- eating for your brain and gut is total welfare

There is a ton of research on brain and gut health and I have included a few papers in the references.
Gastroenterology
Volume 114, Issue 3, March 1998, Pages 559–578
Special Reports and Reviews
Brain-gut axis in health and disease ☆ Qasim Aziz, David G. Thompson

'Hippocrates has been quoted as saying "death sits in the bowels" and "bad digestion is the root of all evil" in 400 B.C. Hawrelak JA, Myers SP. The causes of intestinal dysbiosis: a review. Altern Med Rev 9: 180–197, 2004., showing that the importance of the intestines in human health has been long recognized.'
Gut Microbiota in Health and Disease
Inna Sekirov, Shannon L. Russell, L. Caetano M. Antunes, B. Brett Finlay
Physiological Reviews Published 1 July 2010 Vol. 90 no. 3, 859-904 DOI: 10.1152/physrev.00045.2009

'Hence, our results suggest that the microbial colonization process initiates signaling mechanisms that affect neuronal circuits involved in motor control and anxiety behavior.' vol. 108 no. 7
Rochellys Diaz Heijtz, 3047–3052, doi: 10.1073/pnas.1010529108
Normal gut microbiota modulates brain development and behavior

Rochellys Diaz Heijtza,b,1, Shugui Wangc, Farhana Anuard, Yu Qiana,b, Britta Björkholmd, Annika Samuelssond, Martin L. Hibberdc, Hans Forssbergb,e, and Sven Petterssonc,d,1
Author Affiliations
Edited by Arturo Zychlinsky, Max Planck Institute for Infection Biology, Berlin, Germany, and accepted by the Editorial Board January 4, 2011 (received for review August 11, 2010)

SECTION 1

Listing of conditions and foods that have been successfully treated in the past and may help you

acid reflux
chlorophyll

acne
chlorophyll: cracked chlorella, wheatgrass

allergies
kelp

anti ageing
Cracked chlorella
himalayan pink salt
spirulina
cherry juice
raw sprouted seeds
astaxanthin
maca
matcha
walnuts
goji berries
blueberries

cordyceps sinensis
antiviral
spirulina
watercress
red algae
alkalanising
cracked chlorella
barleygrass
himalayan pink salt
vegetables
allergies
spirulina
goji berries
cacao
alzheimer's
L-Carnitine
cracked chlorella
asthma
sea vegetables
anaemia
chlorophyll and iron
spirulina (very high source)
maca
lemon and citrus
spirulina
goji berries
cacao
antibiotic
watercress
coconut
cacao
cracked chlorella
wheatgrass
red algae
shiitake mushroom
antifungal
coconut
shiitake mushroom
antioxidants

chia seeds
wheatgrass
cherry juice
astaxanthin
chaga
coconut
spirulina
kale
swiss chard
blueberry
cordyceps sinensis

antiviral
sea vegetables
algae
red algae: antiretrovirus
carrageenan
coconut

anxiety
maca

arthritis
cherry juice
sea vegetables
kelp

appetite suppression
matcha

asthma
lemon and citrus
kelp

bacterial infections
chlorophyll: cracked chlorella, wheatgrass
red algae

autism
cracked chlorella

bleeding gums
watercress

blood pressure
cherry juice
matcha

himalayan pink salt
swiss chard
blood sugar
chia seeds
cracked chlorella
wheatgrass
coconut oil
pre-sprouted barley
red algae
blood issues / purification
cracked chlorella
wheatgrass
himalayan pink salt
spirulina
kale
maca
chaga
spirulina
goji berries
watercress
brain issues
leafy greens
goji beries
bone health
kale
raw sprouted seeds
himalayan pink salt
lemon and citrus
bowel issues
wheatgrass
barleygrass
aloe
burns
aloe vera
lemon and citrus
candida
red algae
cancer

cracked chlorella
cherry juice
spirulina (oral)
brassicas: broccoli (breast tumours)
cabbage
cauliflower with turmeric (prostate)
cruciferous vegetables with cir cumin (prostate cancer)
brussels sprouts
kale
watercress (lung, breast, bowel)
raw sprouted seeds
sea vegetables/kelp (breast and intestinal)
chlorophyll containing high levels
cracked chlorella
wheatgrass
sea vegetables (lymphoma)
cancer prevention (combats cancer initiation)
cancer support
chaga (biological response modifier)
bee pollen (prostate)
lemon and citrus
coconut
walnuts (breast, prostate)
goji germanium (anticancer: cervical; liver; lung; testicular; uterus)
cordyceps sinensis (Anti leukaemia, tumour growth cell inhibition in cancer, modulator of systemic immune system)
shiitake mushroom

Cataracts
lemon and citrus

chlorophyll (sources)
spinach
buckwheat sprouts
cracked chlorella
spirulina

cognitive decline
leafy greens: kale
lemon and citrus
walnuts
blueberries

constipation

kale
aloe vera

degenerative diseases
cracked chlorella

deodorant
wheatgrass

depression
maca

diabetes type 2 from trials in women
cherry juice
coconut
walnuts
spirulina

Gastro intestinal tract digestion improvement and issues
cracked chlorella
wheatgrass
himalayan pink salt
aloe vera
spirulina
kale
watercress (protein assimilation)
sea vegetables
chaga

disinfection
cabbage

diverticulosis
brassicas

drug detox
wheatgrass
aloe vera

electrolyte source
coconut water

energy
chia seeds
barleygrass
maca
coconut oil

spirulina
raw sprouted seeds
pre-sprouted barley
astaxanthin
maca
cordyceps sinensis

enzymes
wheatgrass
barleygrass
raw sprouted seeds
chaga
blueberries
swiss chard

epilepsy
L-Carnitine

eyes
watercress
kale
swiss chard
astaxanthin
lemon (cataracts)
goji berries

fertility
wheatgrass (high magnesium levels restore the hormones)
fibre
kale
maca
chlorophyll (improves sperm count)

flu
spirulina
sea vegetables
red algae

free radical scavenging
cracked chlorella
barleygrass
spirulina
cherry juice

food intolerances
spirulina

goitre prevention
himalayan pink salt
gum healing
chlorophyll
coconut
gut flora support
cracked chlorella
kombucha
hair
watercress
hangovers
chlorella
hay fever
chlorophyll
headaches
cabbage (topical)
heart disease
cherry juice
kale
swiss chard
pre-sprouted barley
maca
lemon and citrus
berries: cranberries; blueberries; strawberries
coconut oil
coconut water (cardioprotective)
walnuts
spirulina
cacao
chlorella
goji berries
L-Carnitine
Heavy metal poisoning: mercury and cadmium
cracked chlorella (plus arsenic, aluminium and lead)
wheatgrass
barleygrass
sea vegetables: kelp (so eat with tuna)
red algea

himalayan pink salt
spirulina

herpes simplex
spirulina
sea vegetables
red algae
(restrict nuts: walnuts and peanuts {a legume})

hormones
maca

hypertension
wheatgrass
matcha

hypolipidemic
coconut

immune system support and enhancement
cracked chlorella
wheatgrass
maca
aloe vera
cherry juice
spirulina
swiss chard
chaga fungus (a biological response modifier)
coconut
cordyceps sinensis

impetigo
wheatgrass

inflammation
cherries
blueberries
pomegranates
spirulina
astaxanthin
cherry juice
watercress
sea vegetables/kelp
astaxanthin
matcha
spirulina

goji berries
kelp
cordyceps sinensis

insect repellant
coconut

joint pains
spirulina

leg ulcers
chlorophyll

kidney and adrenal health
goji berries

kidney stone disease
lemon and citrus

leukoplakia
spirulina

libido
himalayan pink salt

liver cleansing and healing
cracked chlorella
wheatgrass
coconut
walnuts

macular degeneration
kale
astaxanthin

magnesium
cacao
cracked chlorella

memory issues
cracked chlorella
coconut
l carnitine

menopause
raw sprouted seeds
sea vegetables
maca
coconut

menstrual issues
sea vegetables
maca
cacao
mental clarity
cracked chlorella
migraine
watercress
maca
walnuts
blueberry
mental health
maca
mineral deficiencies
chia seeds
spirulina
mood swings
maca
mouth health
coconut
chlorophyll (bleeding gums, gingivitis, sore throats, anticancer)
nerve tissue rebuilding in multiple sclerosis
cracked chlorella
nerve and muscle functioning
himalayan pink salt
Neural tube defects
lemon and citrus
cherry juice
sea vegetables
spirulina
neuropathy
matcha
nuclear accidents/radiation
spirulina
cracked chlorella
nutrient absorption improvement
cracked chlorella

himalayan pink salt

obesity
chia seeds
spirulina
astaxanthin
matcha
l carnitine
obesity
cacao

omega 3 source
chia seeds

painkiller
cherryjuice

parasites
wheatgrass

Parkinsons
Cracked chlorella

Pesticides, fungicides
cracked chlorella

Post surgery
lemon and citrus

Premenstrual symptoms
spirulina

prenatal nutrition
spirulina

Prostate enlargement
bee pollen

Protein (Complete)
Chia seeds
spirulina

Radiation poisoning
cracked chlorella

recovery
getting back/restoring your former self/establishing peak performance
cracked chlorella

spirulina
maca
L-Carnitine

scar healing
wheatgrass
bee pollen

sciatica
cracked chlorella

self esteem
maca

seizures
cracked chlorella

sexual function
maca (libido, endurance)

sinusitis
wheatgrass

skin problems
spirulina
watercress
astaxanthin with tocotrienols (vitamin E)
maca
Brussels sprouts (collagen)

skin cancer
spirulina

sleep/insomnia
cherry juice
himalayan pink salt

sore throat
wheatgrass

sperm count
chlorophyll

stress
matcha (reduces cortisol)

sugar craving
swish green juice in your mouth

sunscreen
astaxanthin

thyroid
watercress

tissue repair and regrowth
cracked chlorella

tooth decay/tooth ache
wheatgrass
coconut
shiitake

toxin remover
wheatgrass
coconut water

ulcerative colitis
wheatgrass

ulcers, GIT, Skin
cabbage
chaga
goji berries

Urinary tract
cranberry

wounds
chlorophyll topical
wheatgrass
maca
aloe vera

wrinkles
astaxanthin

THE FOODS DESCRIBED

aloe vera

- Bioactive compounds are stored in the gel in the leaves.
- Antioxidant
- antibacterial
- antiseptic,
- anti inflammatory,
- antiviral
- antifungal
- non allergic
- very good in building up the immune system.
-
- healing of burns (reduces this by 9 days compared to conventional treatment, in trials)

Burns. 2007 Sep;33(6):713-8. Epub 2007 May 17.
The efficacy of aloe vera used for burn wound healing: a systematic review.
Maenthaisong R1, Chaiyakunapruk N, Niruntraporn S, Kongkaew C.

● In trials aloe vera killed streptococcus mutans and candida albicans in the mouth

J Clin Diagn Res. 2014 Oct; 8(10): ZI01–ZI02.
Published online 2014 Oct 20. doi: 10.7860/JCDR/2014/8382.4983
PMCID: PMC4253296
Aloe Vera in Dentistry
G Sujatha,corresponding author1 G Senthil Kumar,2 J Muruganandan,3 and T Srinivasa Prasad4

● Can treat constipation, has a well known laxative effect.
Pharmacology. 1993 Oct;47 Suppl 1:86-97.
Metabolism and pharmacokinetics of anthranoids.
de Witte P1.
But in trials it wasn't shown to be helpful for IBS
Int J Clin Pract. 2006 Sep;60(9):1080-6. Epub 2006 Jun 2.
Randomised double-blind placebo-controlled trial of aloe vera for irritable bowel syndrome.
Davis K1, Philpott S, Kumar D, Mendall M.
● It has found to be useful in type 2 diabetes
Phytomedicine. 1996 Nov;3(3):241-3. doi: 10.1016/S0944-7113(96)80060-2.
Antidiabetic activity of Aloe vera L. juice. I. Clinical trial in new cases of diabetes mellitus.
Yongchaiyudha S1, Rungpitarangsi V, Bunyapraphatsara N, Chokechaijaroenporn O.
Phytomedicine. 1996 Nov;3(3):245-8. doi: 10.1016/S0944-7113(96)80061-4.
Antidiabetic activity of Aloe vera L. juice II. Clinical trial in diabetes mellitus patients in combination with glibenclamide.
Bunyapraphatsara N1, Yongchaiyudha S, Rungpitarangsi V, Chokechaijaroenporn O.
But it has also been to shown affect the liver if taken for prolonged amounts of time.
J Korean Med Sci. 2010 Mar; 25(3): 492–495.
Published online 2010 Feb 17. doi: 10.3346/jkms.2010.25.3.492
PMCID: PMC2826749
● Aloe-induced Toxic Hepatitis

Ha Na Yang,1 Dong Joon Kim,corresponding author1 Young Mook Kim,1 Byoung Ho Kim,1 Kyoung Min Sohn,1 Myung Jin Choi,1 and Young Hee Choi2

On a personal note, I have tested aloe vera and it gave me severe diarrhoea, so build up your use from a gentle amount to reduce this risk.

Amino Acids
L Carnitine
Weightloss:
- L-carnitine transfers long-chain fatty acids, such as triglycerides into mitochondria, where they may be oxidized to produce energy.

L-Carnitine has also been shown to reduce fatigue and serve as an appetite suppressant as well.

It not only will help keep your body from storing fat, but it will increase your aerobic capacity to help you burn more calories.

- Supplementing with l-carnitine can help you increase your strength
- L-carnitine, you can slow down the bone loss process and improve bone micro structural properties by decreasing bone turnover.
- Several clinical trials show that L-carnitine can be used along with conventional treatment for angina to reduce the needs for medicine and improve the ability of those with angina to exercise without chest pain or discomfort. Some studies have determined that taking l-carnitine after a heart attack decreases the chances of suffering another one later. Carnitine has actually been given to help treat people with heart disease.
- L-carnitine helps diabetics by increasing glucose oxidation, glucose storage, as well as glucose uptake.
- L-carnitine helps protect the brain from both age related and stress related damage to the brain

In Alzheimer's disease L carnitine showed a statistically significant difference.

Long-term acetyl-L-carnitine treatment in Alzheimer's disease
A. Spagnoli, MD, U. Lucca, PhD, G. Menasce, MD, L. Bandera, MD, G. Cizza, MD, G. Forloni, PhD, M. Tettamanti, PhD, L. Frattura, MD, P. Tiraboschi, MD, M. Comelli, PhD, U. Senin, MD, A. Longo, MD, A. Petrini, MD, G. Brambilla, MD, A. Belloni, PhD,

C. Negri, MD, F. Cavazzuti, MD, A. Salsi, MD, P. Calogero, MD, E. Parma, MD, M. Stramba-Badiale, MD, S. Vitali, MD, G. Andreoni, MD, M. R. Inzoli, MD, G. Santus, MD, R. Caregnato, MD, M. Peruzza, MD, M. Favaretto, MD, C. Bozeglav, PhD, M. Alberoni, MD, D. De Leo, MD, L. Serraiotto, MD, A. Baiocchi, MD, S. Scoccia, MD, P. Culotta, MD and D. Ieracitano, MD
+SHOW AFFILIATIONS
doi: http://dx.doi.org/10.1212/WNL.41.11.1726
Neurology November 1991 vol. 41 no. 11 1726

astaxanthin

Astaxanthin is a powerful, naturally occurring carotenoid pigment that's found in certain marine plants and animals. Often called "the king of the carotenoids," astaxanthin is recognized as being one of the most powerful antioxidants found in nature. It is of particular significance, because unlike some other types of antioxidants, astaxanthin never becomes a pro-oxidant in the body so it can never cause harmful oxidation.

- fat burning
- increasing energy
- eye health
- anti ageing
- sunscreen taken internally
- wrinkles
- skin condition with vitamin E tocotrienol
- recovery time after exercise, and increased endurance
- antioxidant

barleygrass

- eighteen amino acids including Alanine, Arginine, Aspartic acid, Glutamic acid, Glycine, Histidine, Isoleucine, Leucine, Lysine, Methionine, Phenylalanine, Proline, Serine, Threonine, Tyrosine and Valine.

- All 8 of the essential amino acids are found in Barley grass. Amino acids are the building blocks of proteins, which are the major constituents of our body and are necessary for the continual cell building, cell regeneration and energy production that are necessary for life.

The vitamins found in Barley grass include

- beta-carotene,
- folic acid,
- pantothenic acid,
- vitamin B1,
- vitamin B2.
- vitamin B6
- vitamin C.
- The minerals include:
- potassium,
- calcium.
- magnesium,
- iron,

- copper,
- phosphorus.
- manganese
- zinc.
- plus lots of live enzymes, one of which is the anti ageing enzyme called superoxide dismutase (SOD). SOD aids in digestion and metabolism by helping to disperse vitamins and minerals into the blood stream to be absorbed by the body.
- detoxifies heavy metals

bee pollen

Bee Pollen is flower pollen collected by honeybees and is the insect's primary food source.

Pollen grains, contain concentrations of phytochemicals carotenoids, flavonoids and phytosterols.1

In a placebo-controlled, double-blind clinical trial of 60 men, researchers from the University Hospital of Wales, Cardiff, found pollen extract was an effective treatment for prostate enlargement and prostatitis. In another study, mice with lung cancer survived almost twice as long when treated with pollen extracts compared with untreated controls. Pollen increased the effectiveness of chemotherapy when given simultaneously. Unlike chemotherapy, pollen didn't attack tumours but stimulated immunity.

In trials Honey treatment reduced the average postoperative scar width by nearly two-thirds, and hospitalization duration by half.

blueberries and cranberries

Many of the uses, once thought to be anecdotal, are now the subject of intensive scientific research.

Cranberry juice has been shown clinically to prevent urinary tract infections, (until recently, the effect was thought to be due to acidification of the urine). *Inhibition of bacterial adherence by cranberry juice: potential use for the treatment of urinary tract infections.*
(PMID:6368872) Sobota AE The Journal of Urology [1984, 131(5): 1013-1016]

Research suggests that proanthocyanidins compounds in cranberry inhibit bacterial adherence to the uroepithelium, preventing subsequent colonization and urinary tract infection.

Research on blueberries, originally focused on antioxidant activity, has now expanded to anti-inflammation, and cell signalling. Much research involves the effects of blueberry on age-related mental decline, including cognitive and motor functions.

Increases in functionality have been observed in animal and human trials following consumption of blueberries. Blueberries are known for their broad array of phytochemicals, especially flavonoids,
polyphenols, anthocyanins, micronutrients, and fibre. In epidemiological and clinical studies, these constituents have been associated with improved cardiovascular risk profiles. Human intervention studies using chokeberries, cranberries, blueberries, and strawberries (either fresh, or as juice, or freeze-dried), or purified anthocyanin extracts have demonstrated significant improvements in LDL oxidation, lipid peroxidation, total plasma antioxidant capacity, dyslipidemia, and glucose metabolism. Benefits were seen in healthy test subjects and in those with existing metabolic risk factors. Underlying mechanisms for these beneficial effects are believed to include up-regulation of endothelial nitric oxide synthase, decreased activities of carbohydrate digestive enzymes, decreased oxidative stress, and inhibition of inflammatory gene expression and foam cell formation.

- Data support the recommendation of berries in a heart-healthy diet.

broccoli (brassicas)
- Vitamin C
- sulforaphane
- carotene
- folic acid
- fibre
- minerals, trace elements

Brussels sprouts (brassicas)
- protein (not complete)
- Vitamin C
- supports collagen manufacturer
- betacarotene
- folate
- Vitamin B
- fibre

cabbage (brassicas)
- Vitamin C (more than oranges).
- Essential minerals: potassium; calcium; B1, B2,
- Vitamin E
- Calcium
- Vitamin K
- Raw cabbage (and broccoli and cauliflower) can suppress the thyroid (goitrogenic).
- Cut when needed rather than prepare in advance due to oxidation.
- For ulcers: chopped or juiced cabbage.

cacao
- magnesium: brain power, heart issues
- muscle relaxing in menstrual cramps
- alkalinising
- increases flexibility
- iron: anaemia
- chromium
- manganese
- zinc (increased bioavailability after heavy metal cleanse)
- copper

- Vitamin C
- Omege 6
- Phenylethylamine
- anandamide (found only in cacao) and produced after exercise: the bliss chemical.
- tryptophan (part of the B6 tryptophan serotonin neurotransmitter pathway)
- serotonin
- fibre
- theobromine (a close relative of caffeine): antibacterial and it kills *strep mutans* which causes most cavities is also good for the heart
- Several studies stated that cacao was the number one weightloss food. But not in its processed form with sugar and fat added

cauliflower (brassicas)
- glucosinolates: sulforophane
- thiocyanates (isothiocyanate) which neutralise toxins
- Glutathione transferase, glucuronosyl transferase and quinone reductase are supports to the detox process.

chaga fungus
- cancer prevention and treatment: biological response modifier
- blood vessels
- neuropathy in diabetes
- gastrointestinal health (fights off helicobacter pylori which causes most ulcers)
- antioxidant: polysaccharides; energy, cardiovascular health, blood sugar, and mood enhancement.
- Beta-D-GLucans modulate the immune system, and blood sugar levels (capable of modifying or regulating one or more immune functions and an immunologic adjustment, regulation, or potentiation)
- Betulin and Betulinic acid: cholesterol level
- antioxidant: melanin and polyphenols (highest level of any super food)
- Super oxide dismutase (SOD) are enzymes

chia seeds

- Chia seeds are rich in polyunsaturated fats, especially omega-3 fatty acids. Chia seeds' lipid profile is composed of 60 percent omega-3s, making them one of the richest plant-based sources of these fatty acids -- specifically, of alpha-linolenic acid, or ALA.

- antioxidants that help protect the body from free radicals, ageing and cancer. The high antioxidant profile also helps them have a long shelf life. They last almost two years without refrigeration.

coconut

- Rich in inorganic ions such as potassium (290 mg %), Sodium (42 mg %), Calcium (44 mg %), Magnesium (10 mg %), Potassium (9.2 mg %).
- Coconut flesh reduces tension in the blood vessels, and reduces blood pressure:
- *The ethanolic extract of C. nucifera endocarp has a vasorelaxant and antihypertensive effect, through nitric oxide production in a concentration and endothelium dependent manner, due to direct activation of nitric oxide/guanylate cyclase pathway, stimulation of muscarinic receptors and/or via cyclooxygenase pathway.*
- Fatty acid (%)
- Triacylglycerol composition of virgin coconut oil.
- TAG: triacylglycerol, Cp: caproic, C: capric, La: lauric, M: myristic,
- P: palmitic, O: oleic.
- Antidote effect
- Tender coconut water (TCW) is found to eliminate poisons in case of mineral poisoning, and ameliorate drug induced over dosage toxicity. The TCW aids the quick absorption of drug and makes their peak concentration in the blood easier by its electrolytic effect, which is similar to fructose coupled faster absorption into the cells and body.
- Antioxidant effect
- A free amino acid, L-arginine (30 mg/dL), is present in TCW which significantly reduce the free radical generation[10]. TCW

also contain vitamin C (15 mg/100mL) that significantly reduce lipid peroxidation when introduced in rats[10]. VCO is capable of increasing antioxidant enzymes when supplemented with diets in rats.
- Cardioprotective effect
- Coconut is composed of the fatty acids caprylic acid C-8:0 (8%), capric acid C-10:0 (7%), lauric acid C-12:0 (49%), myristic acid C-14:0 (18%), palmitic acid C-16:0 (8%), stearic acid C-18:0 (2%), oleic acid C-18:1 (6%), linoleum acid C-18:2 (2%).
- It is abundantly (65%) endowed with medium chain saturated fatty acids (MCFAs), which allows them to be directly absorbed from the intestine and sent straight to the liver to be rapidly metabolized for energy production and thus MCFAs do not participate in the biosynthesis and transport of cholesterol.

Coconut water has cardioprotective effects in myocardial infarction due to rich content of mineral ions, especially potassium.

Nevin and Rajamohan showed that coconut lowered total cholesterol, triglycerides, phospholoipids, low density lipoprotein (LDL), very-low density lipoprotein (VLDL), and increased high density lipoprotein (HDL)-cholesterol levels.

Other qualities:
- Electrolyte
- antidote
- antioxidant
- cardioprotective
- anticholesystitic
- antibacterial
- antiatherosclerotic
- hypolipidemic
- anticaries
- antiprotozoal
- anticancer
- immunostimulatory
- antidiabetic
- hepatoprotective
- antifungal
- disinfectant
- insect repellant

collards
great cooked: cooking quadruples bioavailability of protein, triples vitamin C.
similar to kale

cordyceps sinensis (fungus)
- Antioxidant
- Anti leukaemia
- tumour growth cell inhibition in cancer
- modulator of systemic immune system
- antifatigue
- antistress
- anti inflammatory
- anti ageing
- sexual function

'CSE improved the activity of superoxide dismutase, glutathione peroxidase and catalase and lowered the level of lipid peroxidation and monoamine oxidase activity in the aged mice. The study demonstrated that CSE can improve the brain function and antioxidative enzyme activity in mice with d-galactose-induced senescence and promote sexual function in castrated rats. All of these findings suggest that CSE has an antiaging effect'.
Antiaging effect of Cordyceps sinensis extract
Deng-Bo Ji1, Jia Ye1,*, Chang-Ling Li1, Yu-Hua Wang1, Jiong Zhao1 andShao-Qing Cai2

This mushroom tastes really nice. I love it added to my smoothies.

cracked chlorella
- 60% complete protein in free amino acid form (very easily digested)
- 2-7% chlorophyll (which is the highest of any known food)
- Vitamin C
- Vitamin E
- All the known B vitamins (Including B-12 although it's un-absorbable due to B-12 analogues being present as well)
- Calcium (One tbsp. of chlorella contains 320% of the recommended RDA)

- Iron (One tbsp. of chlorella contains 120% of the recommended RDA)
- Magnesium
- Potassium
- Zinc
- Iodine
- Trace minerals
- Omega-3 fatty acids (ALA, DHA and EPA - the last two are often mistakenly thought to only be found in fish and other seafaring animals)
- GLA and other "rare" fatty acids
- Beta-carotene
- Mucopolysaccharides
- Nucleic acids RNA and DNA (Sardines= 0.59% RNA, Chlorella=10% RNA!)
- Enzymes (chlorophyllase and pepsin, the latter helping you digest its high protein content)
- antiageing;
- detox from radiation heavy metal poisoning like mercury and cadmium, pesticides, fertilisers, fungicides,
- mental clarity
- memory improvement from blood purification,
- blood issues,
- for peak performance,
- Liver cleansing,
- Tissue regrowth, and repair,
- immune system enhancement
- free radical scavenging
- speeds up growth of friendly bacteria in the gut, resulting in improved digestion and increased ability to absorb nutrients in your diet.
- Anti cancer.
- against degenerative diseases,
- Rebuilds nerve tissue, in Multiple sclerosis,
- seizures,
- Alzheimers,
- sciatica,
- Parkinsons.
- alkalinising effect on the body.

- chlorella cells include proteins that contain all the amino acids known to be essential for the nutrition of animals and human beings.
- Chlorella also includes many of the vitamins and minerals that support balanced nutrition such as vitamin C, beta-carotene, lutein, thiamine, riboflavin, pyroxidine, niacin, pantothenic acid, folic acid, vitamin B-12, vitamin K, vitamin E, phosphorous, iron, calcium, potassium, magnesium, copper and zinc.
- In addition, chlorella contains omega fatty acids which have been found to promote cardiovascular health.
- Moreover, approximately 5% of each chlorella cell consists of chlorella growth factor (CGF) composed primarily of amino acids, beta-glucan and nucleic acids that are believed to be derived from the nucleus of the algae.

In its natural state, the fibrous cell wall of the chlorella cells prevents the nutrients contained within the chlorella cells from being adequately broken down, digested and absorbed. Thus, chlorella cells will generally pass through the digestive system with little or no benefit. The interior contents of the chlorella cells contain the nutrients that provide the nutritional benefits associated with chlorella, it is necessary to rupture the fibrous cell wall to gain access to the cell contents.

Enzymes must be present in order to utilise the nutrients. people absorb fewer nutrients if there is an inadequate amount of enzymes present in their digestive system. With age, there is greater likelihood that the body may produce fewer enzymes. Enzyme loss may also be attributable due to dietary deficiencies. Although the human body manufactures some enzymes, others are obtained from foods. enzymes are only found in raw foods or in those cooked at temperatures below 118° F. Typically, enzymes begin to perish when cooking temperatures rise above this level. In a diet chronically lacking in raw fruits and vegetables, it may be necessary to include enzymes in supplements that contain natural products rich in plant fibre. Enzymes generally assist in digestion and nutrient assimilation.

Thus, a diet without sufficient quantities of fresh, raw fruits and vegetables can contribute to digestion difficulties when cellulose-rich foods such as chlorella are introduced. As a result,

fermentation and pain may follow. Thus, food enzymes are generally needed to properly digest chlorella.
- Cracked chlorella is best taken with enzymes.

Under fertile growing conditions, each chlorella cell divides into four new cells every 20 to 24 hours. This amounts to about 40 tons per acre annual harvest, as compared to under half a ton of soybeans, or two tons of rice per acre per year. Of course, chlorella contains over 50 percent protein, a much higher percentage than either soybeans or rice. It also contains 19 of 22 amino acids known to be essential to human nutrition.

- Arsenic poisoning has been successfully detoxified with chlorella.

The nutritional profile of chlorella:
- Vitamins
- B1,
- B2,
- B3,
- B6,
- C,
- E,
- pantothenic acid,
- folic acid,
- biotin,
- PABA,
- inositol
- Over 124 micrograms of B12 and over 55,000 IU of vitamin A are found per 100 grams,
- 221 mg of calcium,
- 315 mg of magnesium,
- 130 mg of iron,
- 71 mg of zinc,
- 600 mg of iodine,
- 989 mg of phosphorus.
- Chlorella is the highest known source of chlorophyll, about 2 percent of its weight, and ten times the amount found in alfalfa.
- Chlorophyll is effective in detoxifying the liver and bloodstream, cleansing the bowel, and feeding the friendly bowel flora.
- Iron is more easily absorbed from the bowel in the presence of chlorophyll.

goji berries
- adaptogens: supports adrenals; kidneys and results in more energy, stamina, strength, sexual energy, longevity, protects against liver cancer and hepatitis
- immune function
- alkalinising
- liver protective
- improves blood
- eye sight (xeanthanin and lutein)
- anti-ageing
- nourishes the body and helps it heal
- complete protein (on a par with bee pollen)
- 21 trace minerals
- Not rich in vitamin C
- iron
- beta-sitosterol (anti-inflammatory)
- linoleic acid (essential fat)
- sesquiterpenoids (antiageing)
- tetraterpenoids: xeanthanin and physalin (antioxidant) (2-4 x the antioxidants in blueberries). These protect us from DNA damage and radiation damage.
- polysaccharides
- helps stimulate the body to make Human Growth Hormone
- Longevity
- Beta-carotene (more than carrots) supports thymus gland
- germanium (anticancer: cervical; liver; lung; testicular; uterus)
- choline: brain health
- superoxide dismutase (SOD) is a super antioxidant combats heart disease by fighting oxidised cholesterol
- stomach ulcers
- irritable bowel

For how to use read David Wolfe.
These probiotic features are taken from David Wolfe The Foods and Medicines of the Future
- protection from UV radiation skin damage

I did however find some peer reviewed research on goji berries and problems with hepatitis, one single case of photosensitivity, two cases of anaphylaxis.

Med Clin (Barc). 2012 Sep 22;139(7):320-1. doi: 10.1016/j.medcli.
2012.02.009. Epub 2012 Apr 12.
[Autoimmune hepatitis triggered by consumption of Goji berries].
[Article in Spanish]
Franco M, Monmany J, Domingo P, Turbau M.
Systemic photosensitivity due to Goji berries

Silvia Gómez-Bernal, Laura Rodríguez-Pazos, Francisco Javier García Martínez, Manuel Ginarte, María Teresa Rodríguez-Granados andJaime Toribio
Article first published online: 27 SEP 2011

DOI: 10.1111/j.1600-0781.2011.00603.x
Anaphylaxis Associated With the Ingestion
of Goji Berries (Lycium barbarum)
S Monzón Ballarín,1
 MA López-Matas,2
 D Sáenz Abad,3
 N Pérez-Cinto,1
J Carnés2
1
Allergy Unit. Centro Cinco Villas. CASAR de SALUD. Ejea, Zaragoza, Spain
2
R&D Department. Laboratorios LETI S.L. Tres Cantos, Madrid, Spain 3
Emergency Department, Hospital Clínico Universitario "Lozano Blesa", Zaragoza Spain
However some positive research too:
 Phytochemicals and Health Benefits of Goji Berries

Cesarettin Alasalvar2 andFereidoon Shahidi3
Ying Zhong3, Fereidoon Shahidi3 andMarian Naczk1
Published Online: 24 JAN 2013

DOI: 10.1002/9781118464663.ch6,

Mice drinking goji berry juice (Lycium barbarum) are protected from UV radiation-induced skin damage via antioxidant pathways

Vivienne E. Reeve,*a Munif Allanson,a Sondur Jayappa Arun,a Diane Domanskia and Nicole Paintera
Show Affiliations
Photochem. Photobiol. Sci., 2010,9, 601-607
DOI: 10.1039/B9PP00177H

Himalyan pink salt
- ph balancing
- improves hydration of trace minerals
- improves mineral status of the body
- reduces muscle cramps by improving minerals and hydration
- helps balance blood sugar
- iodine rich
- 80+ minerals and elements including sulphate, magnesium, calcium, potassium, bicarbonate, bromide, borate, strontium, fluoride...
- resulting in
- electrolyte balance
- increased hydration
- water content regulation
- metabolic functioning
- bone strength
- lowers blood pressure
- nutrient absorption in GIT
- prevents goiter
- improve circulation
- dissolves and eliminates toxins
- supports libido
- antiageing
- detoxifies heavy metals
- sinus issues
- respiratory conditions including asthma
- sleep
- arterial health

kale
- Vitamin K for bone formation
- calcium
- lutein and xeanthanin for eye health

- Vitamin C
- sulforaphane
- indoles
- Vitamin B2
- Vitamin B6
- great raw

kelp sea vegetables
- 1.1 milligrams of kelp is the upper limit as too much can cause hyperthyroidism, worsen acne,
- polyphenols
- anticancer: cervix, breast, gastrointestinal
- folate
- magnesium
- fibre
- vitamin B12
- not a safe weight loss food as it can create a hyper-thyroid state
- iodine and selenium: anti breast cancer
- lignans in sea vegetables reduce production of extra oestrogen in fat cells which reduces cancer risk.
- Dulse; hijiki and arame have anti cancer lignin's
- fucoidans in sea vegetables reduces presence of lymphoma cells
- Kelp: fucans (sulphated polysaccharides): anti-inflammatory so good for arthritic conditions, allergies, asthma, autoimmune conditions.

kombucha
- *Kombucha is a fermented tea that is rich in enzymes.*
- *'Kombucha can improve resistance against cancer, prevent cardiovascular diseases, promote digestive functions, stimulate the immune system, reduce inflammatory problems, and can have many other benefits.' Food Research International Volume 33, Issue 6, July 2000, Pages 409–421 Tea, Kombucha, and health: a review*

C. Dufresne, E. Farnworth, Food Research and Development Centre, Agriculture and Agri-Food Canada, 3600 Casavant Blvd. West, Saint-Hyacinthe, QC, Canada J2S 8E3 Available online 12 July 2000

'only a few research studies have shown that Kombucha has in vitro antimicrobial activity and enhances sleep and pain thresholds in rats. Furthermore, Kombucha consumption has proven to be harmful in several documented instances.' Journal of Food Protection®, Number 7, July 2000, pp. 855-986 Kombucha, the Fermented Tea: Microbiology, Composition, and Claimed Health Effects
Authors: Greenwalt, C. J.; Steinkraus, K. H.; Ledford, R. A.
Source: Journal of Food Protection®, Number 7, July 2000, pp. 855-986, pp. 976-981(6)

'The study indicates that rats fed KT for 90 days showed no toxic effects.Subacute (90 days) oral toxicity studies of Kombucha tea.' (PMID:11351863) Vijayaraghavan R , Singh M , Rao PV , Bhattacharya R , Kumar P , Sugendran K , Kumar O , Pant SC , Singh R Defence Research and Development Establishment, Jhansi Road, Gwalior-474002, India. drde@sancharnet.in
Biomedical and Environmental Sciences : BES [2000, 13(4): 293-299]

'The study shows that K-tea has anti-stress and hepato-protective activities.Studies on toxicity, anti-stress and hepato-protective properties of Kombucha tea.' (PMID:11723720) Pauline T , Dipti P , Anju B , Kavimani S , Sharma SK , Kain AK , Sarada SK , Sairam M , Ilavazhagan G , Devendra K , Selvamurthy W Defence Institute of Physiology Allied Sciences, Timarpur, Lucknow Road, Delhi-110054, India.

"Unexplained severe illness (including one death) occurred in two persons in a rural town in northwestern Iowa who had been drinking Kombucha tea daily for approximately 2 months.'
Biomedical and Environmental Sciences : BES [2001, 14(3): 207-213] MMWR Morb Mortal Wkly Rep. 1995 Dec 8;44(48): 892-3, 899-900. Unexplained severe illness possibly associated with consumption of Kombucha tea--Iowa, 1995.
Centers for Disease Control and Prevention (CDC).

'On the basis of these data it was concluded that the largely undetermined benefits do not outweigh the documented risks of kombucha. It can therefore not be recommended for therapeutic use.' Vol. 10, No. 2, 2003 Issue release date: April 2003

Section title: Review Article · Übersichtsarbeit Forsch Komplementärmed Klass Naturheilkd 2003;10:85–87 DOI: 10.1159/000071667) Kombucha: A Systematic Review of the Clinical Evidence
Ernst E. Complementary Medicine, Peninsula Medical School, Universities of Exeter and Plymouth, UK

I have listed various scientific findings for Kombucha. They contrast totally. I conclude that it is up to the individual to research and decide if it is a choice for you.

L-carnitine
- alzheimer's
- memory
- epilepsy in children
- recovery from exercise
- athlete supplementation
- Heart diseases (one meta-analysis showed huge differences between the trial groups and very positively for L-Carnitine)

There is A LOT of research on L-Carnitine and memory and Alzheimer's. I have included a few papers.

leafy greens
- folate for cognitive decline

lemon and citrus
- Phytochemicals:
- monoterpenes
- limonoids (triterpenes)
- flavanoids
- caratenoids
- hydroxycinnamic acid
- Cardiovascular disease
- kidney stone disease
- cancer
- heart disease
- hypertension
- neural tube defects
- anaemia

People with these would benefit:
- smokers
- alcoholics
- burns
- fractures
- fevers
- tuberculosis
- chronic illness
- post surgery
- children
- the elderly
- immunocompromised individuals
- post operative

maca
- Vitamins B, C, E
- Calcium
- zinc
- iron
- magnesium
- phosphorous
- amino acids
- Sexual function: boosts libido and endurance, balances hormones and increases fertility
- menstrual issues, cramps, body pains, menopause flushes, mood swings, depression
- energy increases, more stamina
- blood tonic: restores blood and red blood cells, anaemia, heart disease
- wound healing
- muscle mass
- Not recommended in hormonal cancers: testicular or ovarian
- clears acne and blemishes
- decreases skin sensitivity and extreme temperatures
- anxiety, stress, depression, mood swings have been helped
- increased mental energy and focus

matcha

- caffeine (only have it in the morning)
- antioxidants
- minerals
- vitamins
- heart disease
- cancer
- blood sugar regulation
- anti-ageing
- l-theanine induces relaxation without drowsiness
- reduces cortisol, a stress hormone that drives appetite and increases belly fat
- lowers inflammation (a trigger for premature ageing and disease)
- curbs impulse eating
- lowers blood pressure
- boosts self esteem and compassion
- may contain lead so only one cup daily and do not give to children. But chlorella can chelate all heavy metals, so make sure to have chlorella with your matcha.

pre-sprouted barley
- provides long lasting energy, good nutrition, stamina
- beta-glucan

probiotics
Probiotic cultures naturally occur in certain fermented foods. Below is a list of different strains of probiotic bacteria.

- Bacillus coagulans GBI-30, 6086
- Bifidobacterium animalis subscp. lactis BB-12
- Bifidobacterium longum subsp. infantis 35624
- Lactobacillus acidophilus NCFM
- Lactobacillus paracasei St11
- Lactobacillus johnsonii La1
- Lactobacillus plantarum 299v
- Lactobacillus reuteri ATCC
- Lactobacillus reuteri Protectis
- Saccharomyces boulardii.

- Today, in an era of antibiotic-resistant pathogens and other looming microbial threats, the value of prevention of infection is recognized. Probiotics may play an important role in helping the body protect itself from infection, especially along the colonized mucosal surfaces of the gastrointestinal tract. Probiotic products are available in many different forms worldwide, including pills, powders, foods, and infant formula. In some cases, general health claims are made that cannot be substantiated for the specific strains and levels being used and consumers must therefore beware.
- Probiotics can be bacteria, moulds, yeast. But most probiotics are bacteria. Among bacteria, lactic acid bacteria are more popular. Lactobacillus acidophilus, L. casei, L. lactis, L. helviticus, L. salivarius, L. plantrum, L. bulgaricus, L. rhamnosus, L. johnsonii, L. reuteri, L. fermentum, L. del-brueckii, Streptococcus thermophilus, Enterococcus fae-cium, E. faecalis, Bifidobacterium bifidum, B. breve, B. longum and Saccharomyces boulardii are commonly used bacterial probiotics (Table 1). A probiotic may be made out of a single bacterial strain or it may be a consortium as well12. Probiotics can be in powder form, liquid form, gel, paste, granules or avail-able in the form of capsules, sachets.

Quotes from research (references at the end):
- 'Probiotic strains, especially lactic acid bacteria have a major role to play in the cholesterol lowering mechanism. As the cholesterol level keeps increasing in the serum, it leads to cardiac diseases. These cholesterol levels can be brought down using probiotics.'
- The anticancer benefits of fermented foods were regarded as folklore, with no scientific backing. But, now there is a strong attestation to the importance of Lactobacilli in human nutrition and health, as well as the interrelationship between many dietary factors and cancer. Diets high in animal protein and fat appear to increase the susceptibility to colon cancer, apparently through conversion of procar-cinogens to carcinogens by the intestinal microflora. Fats and fried foods also have been implicated in cancers of breast, prostate and pancreas. The consumption of milk has been negatively correlated to the incidence of gastric cancer and has been postulated to play an important role in prevention of human stomach cancer caused by alkylating agents. On the other

hand, milk consumption has also been positively correlated with the incidence of colon, prostate and breast cancer and has been attributed to in-creased consumption of fat, modification of the intestinal flora by milk components, ingestion of milk hormones and presence of an oncogenic virus or other contaminants in milk.

- It is hypothesized that gut microflora, through the production of carcinogens and tumour promoters, are involved in the aetiology of colorectal cancer. There is some evidence that probiotics can interfere at various stages of the cancer process, such as prevention of DNA damage in the colon by live bacteria, suppression of pre-neoplastic changes in the colon and suppression of colon tumours in animals. Studies on the effect of probiotics consumption on cancer appear to be promising. Animal and in vitro studies indicate that probiotic bacteria may reduce colon cancer risk by reducing the incidence and number of tumours. One clinical study showed an increased recurrence-free period in subjects with bladder cancer. Results, however, are too preliminary to develop specific recommendations on probiotic consumption for preventing cancer in humans.
- Milk is the richest source of calcium and Ca requirement of the body is met only through milk. Hence, a person consuming non-milk diet will naturally develop Ca deficiency, leading to osteoporosis. Birge et al.

(I've included this last quote to show how even in science papers there are assumptions, in this case about calcium and the logic of no dairy consumption leading to calcium deficiency. We know this not to be true. See the super foods listed in this book for sources of calcium).
Peer reviewed papers on menopause are still referring to dairy as a good source of calcium:
(Menopause. 2006 Nov-Dec;13(6):862-77; quiz 878-80.
The role of calcium in peri- and postmenopausal women: 2006 position statement of the North American Menopause Society.)
(Journal of Food Composition and Analysis
Volume 17, Issues 3–4, June–August 2004, Pages 311–320
Papers from the Joint Meeting of the 5th International Food Data Conference and the 27th US National Nutrient Databank Conference

In vitro calcium bioavailability of vegetables, legumes and seeds Achiraya Kamchan, Prapasri Puwastien, , Prapaisri P Sirichakwal, Ratchanee Kongkachuichai) this article mentions non dairy calcium sources but does mention optimum balances. So many research papers talk of dairy or supplementation but not the use of super foods for calcium. Several talk of getting Vitamin D from the sun.

(Progress in Biophysics and Molecular Biology
Volume 92, Issue 1, September 2006, Pages 26–32
UV exposure guidance: A balanced approach between health risks and health benefits of UV and Vitamin D. Proceedings of an International Workshop, International Commission on Non-ionizing Radiation Protection, Munich, Germany, 17-18 October, 2005)

Probiotics as a supplement is one thing, and then there's fermented foods.
There is A LOT of research on fermented foods. Dozens of papers focus on foods from Africa and India. I was looking for information on what they do for us. Do they make a difference. In this trial in India, children who had been very ill with repeated gut infections and were as a result stunted in growth, were given fermented foods for six months and there was much improvement in growth and indeed death from gut infections (when compared to a control group). This is the difference between life or death by use of these.
Nutrition Volume 18, Issue 5, May 2002, Pages 393–396 Applied nutritional investigation Use of fermented foods to combat stunting and failure to thrive Shailee Saran, MSca, Sarath Gopalan, MD, a, , T.Prasanna Krishna, PhDbGoji Berries

raw sprouted seeds
- enzymes for digestion and energy
- buckwheat: chlorophyll
- alfalfa: protein; immunity
- sunflower: protein; immunity
- radish: protein; vitamin c and carotenes, calcium, beta carotene
- broccoli: immunity

red algae
- antiviral
- carrageenan: polysaccharides act as an immunomodulatory agent (Capable of modifying or regulating one or more immune functions and an immunologic adjustment, regulation, or potentiation).
- demontacea: rich in sulphated polysaccharides which improve immune response; antiviral, anticoagulant

shiitake mushroom
There is a lot of research on this mushroom which supports its use as a therapeutic food:
- anti cancer,
- antibacterial,
- anti fungal,
- selenium rich,
- anti caries,

and also a few allergies were reported in a few patients to this mushroom.

spinach
eat some raw and some cooked
- Vitamin C
- Vitamin B1 and B6
- Vitamin E
- Chlorophyll
- carotenes
- folate
- magnesium
- potassium

spirulina
Blue-greenalgae, extremely nutrient dense, with high keels of chlorophyll, vitamins and minerals, and amino acids. Easily digestible, it is fast growing, and doubles its biomass in two to five days. It grows well where nothing else grows and yields over 20 times the protein that soybeans do and 400 times the beef protein yield (per equivalent land space).

- Spirulina contains 10 times more betacarotene than carrots, GLA, omega 6.

heavy metal detox
- diabetes: more effective in some trials than metformin
- muscle strength and (in some trials) endurance.
- anaemia
- immune function
- allergic rhinitis
- reduces blood pressure
- oral cancers

In a study of 37 individuals with type 2 diabetes, 8 grams of spirulina per day significantly reduced markers of oxidative damage. It also increased levels of antioxidant enzymes in the blood

beneficial in trials for diabetes and heart disease (in dosages ranging from 2-8 grams a day).
- A single tablespoon (7 grams) of dried spirulina powder contains:
- Protein: 4 grams.
- Vitamin B1 (Thiamin): 11% of the RDA.
- Vitamin B2 (Riboflavin): 15% of the RDA.
- Vitamin B3 (Niacin): 4% of the RDA.
- Copper: 21% of the RDA.
- Iron: 11% of the RDA.
- magnesium,
- potassium
- manganese
- small amounts of almost every other nutrient that we need.

This is coming with only 20 calories, and 1.7 grams of digestible carbohydrate.

Gram for gram, this means that spirulina may literally be the single most nutritious food on the planet

It is often claimed that spirulina contains vitamin B12, but this is false. It contains pseudovitamin B12, which has not been shown to be effective in humans

swiss chard
- potassium for blood pressure
- vitamins C K E

- carotenes
- antioxidants

walnuts
- l-Arginine (good the the heart and blood pressure) but limit intake if you have herpes as high levels of arginine can deplete lysine which triggers it
- plant-based omega-3 fat alpha-linolenic acid (ALA), which is anti-inflammatory and may prevent the formation of pathological blood clots.

Research shows that people who eat a diet high in ALA are less likely to have a fatal heart attack and have a nearly 50 percent lower risk of sudden cardiac death.

Eating four walnuts a day has been shown to significantly raise blood levels of heart-healthy ALA
walnut consumption supports healthful cholesterol levels.

Research showed that eating just one ounce of walnuts a day may decrease cardiovascular risk, and among those at high cardiovascular risk, increased frequency of nut consumption significantly lowers the risk of death.
- Antioxidants: quinone; juglone; the tannin tellimagrandin; and the flavonol morin.
- Walnut polyphenols may prevent chemically induced liver damage.
- Walnut polyphenols had the best efficacy among the nuts tested and also the highest lipoprotein-bound antioxidant activity: they reduce inflammation without weight gain.
- weightloss

walnuts eaten daily significantly improve sperm quality, including vitality, motility, and morphology
Walnuts contain neuroprotective compounds:
- vitamin E,
- folate,
- melatonin,
- omega-3 fats,
- antioxidants.

Research shows walnut consumption may support brain health, including increasing inferential reasoning in young adults.

High-antioxidant foods like walnuts *'can decrease the enhanced vulnerability to oxidative stress that occurs in ageing," "increase health span,'* and also *'enhance cognitive and motor function in ageing.'*

watercress
only consume raw
- Vitamin C
- Calcium
- folate
- betacarotene
- phenylethyl isothiocyanate
- iodine (thyroid function)
- high sulphur content has important role in protein absorption, blood purification, and healthy hair and skin
- germanium: antiviral, detoxifying, oxygenating, strengthening, intercellular communication
- adaptogen: healths body achieve optimum health possible

wheatgrass
- crude chlorophyll which is non toxic at all levels
- contains all minerals known to man, and vitamins A, B-complex, C, E, I and K. It is extremely rich in protein, and contains 17 amino acids
- Chlorophyll contains enzymes and super-oxide dismutase (SOD) which is anti ageing
- arrests unfriendly bacteria
- contains over 100 elements
- topical skin use: eczema; itching; insect bites and stings
- congested head colds: it dires mucous
- neutralises toxins
- clears drugs from the body
- antiseptic
- heals wounds
- leg ulcers
- dissolves scars in the lungs
- energy

- full spectrum of vitamins and minerals
- detergent
- deodorant
- toothache (hold in the mouth for several minutes)
- sore throat (gargle)
- arthritis (topical)
- constipation (high in magnesium)
- blood disorders
- removes heavy metals
- gluten free
- strength and stamina
- 'This plant is believed to have many nutritional values; it has been shown to have anti-inflammatory, antioxidant, anti-carcinogenic, immunomodulatory, laxative, astringent, diuretic, antibacterial and anti-aging properties. Its use in acidity, colitis, kidney malfunctions, atherosclerosis and swelling has been shown to be beneficial. Wheatgrass juice helps in building red blood cells and stimulates healthy tissue cell growth.'

RESEARCH PAPERS AND REFERENCES

Here follows a mixture of actual references and loads of research papers for your perusal.

aloe vera

PDR for herbal medicines. ed.1. Montvale, NJ: Medical Economics Company; 1998. p. 631.

Akinvele BO, Odiyi AC. Comparative study of the vegetative morphology and the excisting taxonomic status of Aloe vera L. Journal of Plant Sciences. 2007;2(5):558–63.

Gong M, Wang F, Chen Y. Study on application of arbuscular – mycorrhizas in growing seedings of Aloevera.Zhang vao cai= Zhangvaocai. Journal of Chinese Medicinal Materials. 2002;25(1): 1–3. [PubMed]

Vogler BK, Ernst E. Aloe vera: A systemic review of its clinical effectiveness. Br J Gen Pract. 1999;49:823–28. [PMC free article] [PubMed]

Atherton P. Aloe vera revisited. Br J Phytotherapy. 1998;4:176–83.
Hayes SM. Lichen planus- Report of successful treatment with aleo vera. Gen Dent. 1999;47:268–72. [PubMed]

Yamaguchi I, Mega N, Sanada H. Components of the gel Aloevera (L) burm. F. Biosci Biotechnol Biochem. 1993;57:1350–52. [PubMed]

Heggers JP, Pineless GR, Robson MC. Dermaide aloe/aloevera gel: Comparision of the antimicrobial effects. J Am Med Technol. 1979;41:293–94.

Heggers JP, Kucukcelibi A, Stabenou CJ, Ko F, Broemeling LD, Robson MC, Winters WD. Wound healing effects of aloe gel and other topical antibacterial agents in rat skin. Phytotherapy Res. 1995;9:455–57.

Sydiskis RJ, Owen DG, Lohr JL, Rosler KH, Blomster RN. Inactivation of enveloped viruses by anthraquinones extracted from plants. Antimicrob agents Chemother. 1991;35:2463–66. [PMC free article] [PubMed]

Vazquez B, Avila G, Segura D, Escalante B. Antiinflammatory activity of extractracts from Aloevera gel. J Ethnopharmacol. 1996;55(1):69–75. [PubMed]

Meadows TP. Aloe as a humectant in new skin preparations. Cosmetic toiletries. 1980;95:51–56.
Davis RH, Leitner MG, Russo JM, Byrne ME. Antiinflammatory activity of aloevera agaist a spectrum of irritants. J Am Podiat Med Assoc. 1989;79:263–76. [PubMed]

Davis RH, Donato JJ, Hartman GM, Hass RC. Anti-inflammatory and wound healing activity of a growth substance in aloe vera. J Am Podiatr Med Assoc. 1994;84(2):77–81. [PubMed]

Villalobos OJ, Salazar CR, Sánchez GR. Efecto de un enjuague bucal compuesto de aloe vera en la placa bacterianae einflammation gingival. Acta Odontol Venez. 2001;39(2):16–24.

Sílvia Morgana Araújo de Oliveira1, Ticiana Carneiro Torres, Sérgio Luís da Silva Pereira, Olívia Morais de Lima Mota, Márlio Ximenes. Carlos effect of a dentifrice containing aloe vera on plaque and gingivitis control. A double-blind clinical study in humans. J Appl Oral Sci. 2008;16(4):293–99. [PubMed]

Bhatt Geetha, Praveen K, Dodwad Vidya. Aloe vera: Nature's soothing healer to periodontal disease. J of Indian Soc Periodontology. 2011;15(3):205–09. [PMC free article] [PubMed]

Lee SS, Zhang W, Li Y. The antimicrobial potential of 14 natural herbal dentifrices: Results of an in vitro diffusion method study. J Am Dent Assoc. 2004;135(5):1133–41. [PubMed]
Wynn RL. Aloe vera gel : Update for dentistry. Gen Dent. 2005;53(1):6–9. [PubMed]

George Dilip, Bhatt Sham S, Antony Beena. Tooth gel : healing power of Aloe vera proves beneficial to teeth and gums. General Dentistry. 2009:238–41. [PubMed]

Poor MR, Hall JE, Poor AS. Reduction in the incidence of alveolar ostetitis in patients treated with the SaliCept Patch, containing acemannan hrdrogel. J Oral Maxillofac Surg. 2002;60:374–79. [PubMed]

Sudworth R. Philadelphia: Positive Health Publications Ltd; 2002. The use of Aloe Vera in Dentistry.

Salazar-Sanchez N, Lopez-Jornet P, Camacho-Alonso F, Sanchez-Siles M. Efficacy of topical Aloe vera in patients with oral lichen planus: a randomized double-blind study. J Oral Pathol Med. 2010;39(10):735–40. [PubMed]
New products and focus on infection control and surgery design. British Dent J. 2012;212(1):47.

Yagi A, Kabash A, Okamura N, Haraguchi H, Moustafa SM, Khalifa TI. Antioxidant, free radical scavenging and anti inflammatory effects of aloesin derivatives in aloe vera. Planta Med. 2002;68:957–60. [PubMed]

Hu Y, Xu J, Hu Q. Evaluation of antioxidant potential of aloe vera. (Aloe barbadensis Miller) extracts. J Agric Food Chem. 2003;51:7788–91. [PubMed]

"Changes induced by Chlorella on the Body Weight and incidence of Colds Among Naval Trainees." Midorf, 1, 1970.

Umexawa, et al. "Physico-Chemical and Biological Properties of Chron A, an Acid Polysaccharide Originating from Chlorella." Chemotherapy, Vol. 30, No. 9, Sept 1982.

Yamagishi, Yoshio. "The Treatment of Peptic Ulcers by Chlorella." Nihon III Shimpo. No 1997, 1962.

Yamaguchi, Shimizu, et al. "Immuno Modulation by Single Cellular Algae (Chlorella Pyrenoldosa) and Anti-tumor Activities for Tumor-Bearing Mice," a paper presented at the 3rd International Congress of Developmental and Comparative Immunology, Reims, France, July 1985.

Yamada, Yoshio, et al. "School Children's Growth and the Value of Chlorella." Nihon III shimpo, No. 2196, 1988.

Frank, Dr. Benjamin, "Dr. Frank's No-Aging Diet." B of A Communications Co., Baton Rouge, LA (1981).

bee pollen

Markham KR, Campos M. 7- and 8-o-methylherbacetin-3-o-sophorosides from bee pollens and some structure/activity observations. Phytochemistry 1996;43:763-7.

Buck AC, et al. Treatment of outflow tract obstruction due to benign prostatic hyperplasia with the pollen extract Cernilton, a double-blind, placebo-controlled study. Br J Urol 1990;66:398-404.

Furusawa E, et al. Antitumor potential of pollen extract on Lewis lung carcinoma implanted intraperitoneally in syngenic mice. Phytother Res 1995;9:255-9.

Ceglecka M, et al. Effect of pollen extracts on prolonged poisoning of rats with organic solvents. Phytother Res 1991:5;245-9.

Subrahmanyam M. Topical application of honey in treatment of burns. Br J Surg 1991;78:497-8.

Al-Waili NS, Saloom KY. Effects of topical honey on post-operative wound infections due to gram-positive and gram-negative bacteria following caesarean sections and hysterectomies. Eur J Med Res 1999;4:126-30.

Molan PC. The antibacterial activity of honey, Part 1 and Part 2. Bee World 1992;73:5-76.

Allen K, et al. A survey of the antibacterial activity of some New Zealand honeys. J Pharm Pharmacol 1991;43:817-22.

Somal NA, et al. Susceptibility of Helicobacter pylori to the antibacterial activity of manuka honey. J Royal Soc Med 1994;87:9-12.

Frankel S, et al. Antioxidant capacity and correlated characteristics of 14 unifloral honeys. J Apic Res 1998;37:27-31.

Burdock GA. Review of the biological properties of propolis and toxicity of bee propolis (propolis). Food Chem Toxicol 1998;36:347-63.

Bankova VS, et al. Isopentyl cinnamates from poplar buds and propolis. Phytochemistry 1989;28:871-3.

Duke JA, et al. U.S. Dept. of Agriculture Phytochemical and Ethnobotanical Data Base (http://www.ars-grin.gov/duke/) 1999.

Chinthalapally VR, et al. Inhibitory effect of caffeic acid esters on azoxymethane-induced biochemical changes and aberrant crypt foci formation in rat colon. Canc Res 1993;53:4182-8.

Mirzoeva OK, Calder PC. The effect of propolis and its components on eicosanoid production during the inflammatory response. Prostagland Leukot Essent Fatty Acid 1996;55:441-9.

Greenaway W, et al. The composition and plant origins of propolis: a report of work at Oxford. Bee World 1990;71:107-18.

Cheng PC, Wong G. Honey bee propolis: prospects in medicine. Bee World 1996;77:8-14.

Krell R. Value-added products from bee keeping. FAO Agricultural Services Bulletin 124; 1996.

Ghisalberti EL. Propolis: a review. Bee World 1979;60:59-84.

Amoros M, et al. Comparison of the anti-herpes simplex virus activities of propolis and 3-methyl-but-2-enyl caffeate. J Nat Prod 1994;57:644-7.

Krol W, et al. Inhibition of neutrophils chemiluminescence by ethanol extracts of propolis (EEP) and its phenolic components. J Ethnopharm 1996;55:19-25.

Bloodworth BC, et al. Liquid chromatographic determination of trans-10-hydroxy-2-decenoic acid content of commercial products containing royal jelly. J AOAC Int. 1995;78:1019-23.

Ziboh VJ. The significance of polyunsaturated fatty acids in cutaneous biology. Lipids 1996;31:S249-53.

Lecker G, et al. Components of royal jelly II: the lipid fraction, hyrocarbons and sterols. J Apic Res 1982;21:178-84.

Iannuzzi J. Royal jelly: mystery food, in three parts. Am Bee J 1990;8:532-4, 587-9, 659-62.

Vittek J. Effect of royal jelly on serum lipids in experimental animals and humans with atherosclerosis. Experientia 1995;51:927-35.

berries
C. Leigh Broadhurst, Ph.D., heads 22nd Century Nutrition, a nutrition/scientific consulting firm, and is a visiting scientist at a government nutrition research laboratory.
Bandura, A. 1986. Social foundation of thought and action: a social cognitive theory. Englewood Cliffs, NJ, USA, Prentice-Hall.

Block, G., Patterson, B. & Subat, A. 1992. Fruit, vegetable, and cancer prevention: a review of the epidemiological evidence. Nutrition and cancer, 18(1): 1-29.

Bloom, H. 1998. Determinants of plasma homocysteine. American Journal of Clinical Nutrition, 67: 188-189.

Carpenter, K. 1986. The history of scurvy and vitamin C. Cambridge, UK, Cambridge University Press.

Centers for Disease Control and Prevention. 1992. Recommendations for the use of folic acid to reduce the number of cases of spina bifida and other neural tube defects. Morbidity and Mortality Weekly Report (MMWR), 41(RR-14): 1-7 (Review).

Cleveland, L., Goldman, J. & Borrud, L. 1996. Results from USDA's 1994 Continuing Survey of Food Intakes by Individuals and 1994 Diet and Health Knowledge Survey, p. 1-68. Riverdale, Md., USA, USDA.

Contento, I. 1995. The effectiveness of nutrition education and implications for nutrition education, policy, programs, and research: a review of research. J. Nutr. Educ., 27: 277-418.

Fleming, D., Jacques, P., Dallal, G., Tucker, K., Wilson, P. & Wood, R. 1998. Dietary determinants of iron stores in a free living elderly population: The Framingham Heart Study. American Journal of Clinical Nutrition, 67: 722-733.

FMI. 1998. Trends in the United States. Washington, DC, Food Marketing Institute.

cacao
Contemporary Reviews in Cardiovascular Medicine
Cocoa and Cardiovascular Health
Roberto Corti, MD*; Andreas J. Flammer, MD*; Norman K. Hollenberg, MD, PhD; Thomas F. Lüscher, MD

citrus

Gershoff, S. 1993. Vitamin C (ascorbic acid): new roles, new requirements? Nutrition Reviews, 51(11): 313-326.

Gutherie, H. & Picciano, M. 1995. Human nutrition. St Louis, MO, USA, Mosby.

Harats, D., Chevion, S., Nahir, M., Norman, Y., Sagee, O. & Berry, B. 1998. Citrus fruit supplementation reduces lipoprotein oxidation in young men ingesting a diet high in saturated fat: presumptive evidence for an interaction between vitamins C and E in vivo. American Journal of Clinical Nutrition, 67: 240-245.

Hatch, G. 1995. Asthma, inhaled oxidants, and dietary antioxidants. American Journal of Clinical Nutrition, 61(suppl): 625S-630S.

Jacques, P., Taylor, A., Hankinson, S., Willet, W., Mahnken, B., Lee, Y., Vaid, K. & Lahav, M. 1997. Long-term vitamin C supplement use and prevalence of early age-related lens opacities. American Journal of Clinical Nutrition, 66: 911-916.

Nestle, M. et al., 1998. Behavioral and social influences on food choice. Nutrition Reviews, 56(5, Part II): S50-S74.

New, S., Bolton-Smith, C., Grubb, D. & Reid, D. 1997. Nutritional influences on bone mineral density; a cross-sectional study in premenopausal women. American Journal of Clinical Nutrition, 65: 1831-1839.

Ortega, R., Requejo, A., Andres, P., Lopez-Sobaler, A., Quintas, M., Redondo, R., Navia, B. & Rivas, T. 1997. Dietary intake and cognitive function in a group of elderly people. American Journal of Clinical Nutrition, 66: 803-809.

Putnam, J. & Allshouse, J. 1997. Food consumption, prices, and expenditures. Washington, DC, Economic Research Service, USDA.

Steinmetz, K. & Potter, J. 1991. Vegetables, fruit, and cancer, II. Mechanisms. Cancer Causes and Control, 2: 427-442.

Tucker, K., Selhub, J., Wilson, P. & Rosenberg, I. 1996. Dietary pattern relates to plasma folate and homocysteine concentrations in the Framingham Heart Study. Journal of Nutrition, 126: 3025-3031.

United States National Academy of Sciences, Food and Nutrition Board. 1989. Diet and health: implications for reducing chronic disease risk. Washington, DC, National Academy Press.

United States National Academy of Sciences, Food and Nutrition Board. 1990. Recommended dietary allowances. Washington, DC, National Academy Press. Tenth ed.

USDA. 1996. Dietary Guidelines for Americans. Washington, DC, Government Printing Office.

USDA. 1997. World Horticultura; trade and US export. Washington, DC.

Whitney, E. & Rolfes, S. 1999. Understanding nutrition. Belmont, Ca., USA, West/Wadsworth. Eighth ed. (ed. W. Rolfes).
Blueberries Decrease Cardiovascular Risk Factors in Obese Men and Women with Metabolic Syndrome1,2,3
Arpita Basu4,*, Mei Du6, Misti J. Leyva5, Karah Sanchez4, Nancy M. Betts4, Mingyuan Wu6, Christopher E. Aston5, and Timothy J. Lyons5,6
Howell, A.B. (2009). UPDATE ON HEALTH BENEFITS OF CRANBERRY AND BLUEBERRY. Acta Hortic. 810, 779-785
DOI: 10.17660/ActaHortic.2009.810.104
http://dx.doi.org/10.17660/ActaHortic.2009.810.104

Howell, A.B. (2009). UPDATE ON HEALTH BENEFITS OF CRANBERRY AND BLUEBERRY. Acta Hortic. 810, 779-785
DOI: 10.17660/ActaHortic.2009.810.104
http://dx.doi.org/10.17660/ActaHortic.2009.810.104
Berries: emerging impact on cardiovascular health

Arpita Basu , Michael Rhone and Timothy J Lyons
Department of Nutritional Sciences, 301 Human Environmental Sciences, Oklahoma State University (OSU), Stillwater, Oklahoma, USA
Harold Hamm Oklahoma Diabetes Center, University of Oklahoma Health Sciences Center (OUHSC), Oklahoma City, Oklahoma, USA

↵A Basu, Nutritional Sciences, 301 Human Environmental Sciences, Oklahoma State University, Stillwater, OK 74078-6141, USA. E-mail: arpita.basu@okstate.edu, Phone: +1-405-744-4437, Fax: +1-405-744-1357.

coconut

E Chan, CR Elevitch
Species profiles for Pacific island agroforestry, 2006. [Online] Available from: www.traditionaltree.org [Accessed on November 03, 2010].

NMCE
Report on copra, National Multi-commodity Exchange of India Limited (2007), pp. 1–14

CS Dayrit
The truth about coconut oil: The drugstore in a bottle, Anvil Publishing, Inc, Philippines (2005)

L Vestlund
The healing power of organic virgin coconut oil, 2009. [Online] Available from: http://cocofat.com/virgin-coconut-oil-vco-r.html [Accessed on November 12, 2010].

United States Department of Agriculture (USDA)
National nutrient database for standard reference, Nuts, coconut water, 2008. [Online]
Available from: http://www.nal.usda.gov/fnic/foodcomp/cgi-bin/list_nut_edit.pl/ [Accessed on December 8, 2009].

WJWH Yong, L Ge, YF Ng, SN Tan
The chemical composition and biological properties of coconut (Cocos nucifera L.)
Molecules, 14 (2009), pp. 5144–5164

Bawalan DD, Chapman KR. Virgin coconut oil: Production manual for micro-and village-scale processing. FAO Regional Office for

Asia and the Pacific, Bangkok: Food and Agriculture Organization of the United Nations; 2006, p. 1-112.

AM Marina, YB Che Man, SAH Nazimah, I Amin
Chemical properties of virgin coconut oil
J Am Oil Chem Soc, 86 (2009), pp. 301–307

GS Effiong, PE Ebong, EU Eyong, AJ Uwah, UE Ekong
Amelioration of chloramphenicol induced toxicity in rats by coconut water
J Appl Sc Res, 6 (4) (2010), pp. 331–335

AL Loki, T Rajamohan
Hepatoprotective and antioxidant effect of tender coconut water on CCl4 induced liver injury in rats
Indian J Biochem Biophy, 40 (2003), pp. 354–357

GR Bankar, PG Nayak, P Bansal, P Paul, KSR Pai, RK Singla, et al.
Vasorelaxant and antihypertensive effect of Cocos nucifera Linn. endocarp on isolated rat thoracic aorta and DOCA salt-induced hypertensive rats
J Ethnopharmacol (2010) http://dx.doi.org/10.1016/j.jep.2010.11.047

KG Nevin, T Rajamohan
Virgin coconut oil supplemented diet increases the antioxidant status in rats
Food Chem, 99 (2005), pp. 260–266

MG Enig
Coconut: In support of good health in the 21st Century, 2004. [Online]
Available from: http://www.apcc.org.sg/special.htm [Accessed on December 27, 2010].

KG Nevin, T Rajamohan
Beneficial effects of virgin coconut oil on lipid parameters and in vitro LDL oxidation
Clin Biochem, 37 (2004), pp. 830–835

KG Nevin, T Rajamohan
Influence of virgin coconut oil on blood coagulation factors, lipid levels and LDL oxidation in cholesterol fed Sprague-Dawley rats
Eur e-J Clin Nutr Metabol (2007), pp. e1–e8

H Müller, AS Lindman, A Blomfeldt, I Seljeflot, JI Pedersen
A diet rich in coconut oil reduces diurnal postprandial variations in circulating tissue plasminogen activator antigen and fasting lipoprotein(a) compared with a diet rich in unsaturated fat in women
J Nutr, 133 (11) (2003), pp. 3422–3427

AI Ibrahim, MT Obeid, MJ Jouma, GA Moasis, WL Al-Richane, I Kindermann, et al.
Detection of herpes simplex virus, cytomegalovirus and Epstein-Barr virus DNA in atherosclerotic plaques and in unaffected bypass grafts
J Clin Virol, 32 (1) (2005), pp. 29–32

D Esquenazi, MD Wigg, MM Miranda, HM Rodrigues, JB Tostes, S Rozental, et al.
Antimicrobial and antiviral activities of polyphenolics from Cocos nucifera Linn. (Palmae) husk fiber extract
Res Microbiol, 153 (10) (2002), pp. 647–652

S Mini, T Rajamohan
Influence of coconut kernel protein on lipid metabolism in alcohol fed rats
Indian J Exp Biol, 42 (1) (2004), pp. 53–57

V Eckarstein, JR Noter, G Assmann
High density lipoproteins and atherosclerosis. Role of cholesterol efflux and reverse cholesterol transport
Arterioscler Thromb Vasc Biol, 21 (2002), pp. 13–27

MA Abate, TL Moore
Monooctanoin use for gallstone dissolution
Drug Intell Clin Pharm, 19 (1985), pp. 708–713

Daftary GV, Pai SA, Shanbhag GN. Stable emulsion compositions for intravenous administration having preservatie efficacy. United States Patent Application 20080262084. (10/23/2008).

AR Oyi, JA Onaolapo, RC Obi
Formulation and antimicrobial studies of coconut (Cocos nucifera Linne) Oil
Res J Appl S Eng Tech, 2 (2) (2010), pp. 133–137

H Thormar, H Hilmarsson, G Bergsson
Stable concentrated emulsions of the 1-monoglyceride of capric acid (monocaprin) with microbicidal activities against the food-borne bacteria Campylobacter jejuni, Salmonella spp., and Escherichia coli
Appl Environ Microbiol, 72 (1) (2006), pp. 522–526

H Thormar, H Hilmarsson
The role of microbicidal lipids in host defense against pathogens and their potential as therapeutic agents
Chem Phy lipids, 150 (1) (2007), pp. 1–11

S Mandal, MD Mandal, NK Pal, K Saha
Synergistic anti-Staphylococcus aureus activity of amoxicillin in combination with Emblica officinalis and Nymphae odorata extracts
Asian Pacific J Trop Med, 3 (2010), pp. 711–714

S Mandal, M Mandal, NK Pal
Antibacterial potential of Azadirachta indica seed and Bacopa monniera leaf extracts against multidrug resistant Salmonella enterica serovar Typhi isolates
Archives Med Sci, 3 (2007), pp. 14–18

Obi RC, Oyi AR, Onaolapo JA. Antimicrobial activities of coconut (Cocos nucifera Linne) oil. 2nd Annual National Scientific Conference. Ahmadu Bello University, Zaria, Nigeria: National Association of Pharmacists in Academia; 2005, p. 81.

DS Alviano, KF Rodrigues, SG Leitão, ML Rodrigues, ML Matheus, PD Fernández, et al.

Antinociceptive and free radical scavenging activities of Cocos nucifera L. (Palmae) husk fiber aqueous extract
J Ethnopharmacol, 92 (2004), pp. 269–273

WS Alviano, DS Alviano, CG Diniz, AR Antoniolli, CS Alviano, LM Farias, et al.
In vitro antioxidant potential of medicinal plant extracts and their activities against oral bacteria based on Brazilian folk medicine
Arch Oral Biol, 53 (2008), pp. 545–552

JB Taheri, FW Espineli, H Lu, M Asayesh, M Bakshi, MR Nakhostin
Antimicrobial effect of coconut flour on oral microflora: An in vitro study
Res J Biol Scs, 5 (6) (2010), pp. 456–459

W Barnabé, T de Mendonça Neto, FC Pimenta, LF Pegoraro, JM Scolaro
Efficacy of sodium hypochlorite and coconut soap used as disinfecting agents in the reduction of denture stomatitis, Streptococcus mutans and Candida albicans
J Oral Rehabil, 31 (5) (2004), pp. 453–459

AL Agero, VM Verallo-Rowell
A randomized double-blind controlled trial comparing extra virgin coconut oil with mineral oil as a moisturizer for mild to moderate xerosis
Dermatitis, 15 (2004), pp. 109–116

BG Carpo, VM Verallo-Rowell, JJ Kabara
Novel antibacterial activity of monolaurin compared with conventional antibiotics against organisms from skin infections: an in vitro study
Drugs Dermatol, 6 (10) (2007), pp. 991–998

VM Verallo-Rowell, KM Dillague, BS Syah-Tjundawan
Novel antibacterial and emollient effects of coconut and virgin olive oils in adult atopic dermatitis
Dermatitis, 19 (6) (2008), pp. 308–315

Arora R, Chawla R, Marwah R, Arora P, Sharma RK, Kaushik V, et al. Potential of complementary and alternative medicine in preventive management of novel H1N1 flu (Swine flu) pandemic: thwarting potential disasters in the Bud. Evid-Based Complement Alternat Med 2011. doi:10.1155/2011/586506.

Z Rihakova, V Filip, M Plockova, J Smidrkal, R Cervenkova
Inhibition of Aspergillus niger DMF 0801 by monoacylglycerols prepared from coconut oil
Czech J Food Sci, 20 (2002), pp. 48–52

DO Ogbolu, AA Oni, OA Daini, AP Oloko
In vitro antimicrobial properties of coconut oil on Candida sp. in Ibadan, Nigeria
J Med Food, 10 (2) (2007), pp. 384–387

RR Mendonca-Filho, IA Rodrigues, DS Alviano, ALS Santos, RMA Soares, CS Alviano, et al.
Leishmanicidal activity of polyphenolic-rich extract from husk fiber of Cocos nucifera Linn. (Palmae)
Res Microbiol, 155 (2004), pp. 136–143

J Sosnowska, H Balslev
American palm ethnomedicine: A meta-analysis
J Ethnobiol Ethnomed, 5 (2009), p. 43

PR Koschek, DS Alviano, CS Alviano, CR Gattas
The husk fiber of Cocos nucifera L. (Palmae) is a source of antineoplastic activity
Braz J Med Biol Res, 40 (2007), pp. 1339–1343

H Winarsi, Hernayanti, A Purwanto
Virgin coconut oil (VCO) enriched with Zn as immunostimulator for vaginal Candidiasis patient
Hayati J Biosc, 15 (4) (2008), pp. 135–139

AG Vigila, X Baskaran
Immunomodulatory effect of coconut protein on cyclophosphamide induced immune suppressed Swiss Albino mice
Ethnobot Leaflets, 12 (2008), pp. 1206–1212

G Salil, KG Nevin, T Rajamohan
Arginine rich coconut kernel protein modulates diabetes in alloxan treated rats
Chemico-Biol Interact (2010) http://dx.doi.org/10.1016/j.cbi.2010.10.015

J Kneiflova, M Slosarek, V Melicherciková, J Paríkova
Microbicidal effect of Lautercide, a new disinfectant
Cesk Epidemiol Mikrobiol Imunol, 41 (6) (1992), pp. 355–361

Dautel H, Hilker M, Kahl O, Siems K. Verwendung von Dodecansäureals Zeckenrepellent. Patentschrift DE 199 25 838 C 1. Deutsches Patent- und Markenamt. (01.03.2001).

M Sylla, L Konan, JM Doannio, S Traore
Evaluation of the efficacity of coconut (Cocos nucifera), palm nut (Eleais guineensis) and gobi (Carapa procera) lotions and creams in indivirual protection against Simulium damnosum s.l. bites in Cote d'Ivoire
Bull Soc Pathol Exot, 96 (2) (2003), pp. 104–109

CA Robeerto
Cocobiodiesel. Coconut methyl ester (CME) as petrodiesel quality enhancer, Dept. Agr. Philippine Coconut Authority (2001), pp. 1–37

N Radenahmad, U Vongvatcharanon, B Withyachumnarnkul, JR Connor
Serum levels of 17β-estradiol in ovariectomized rats fed young-coconut-juice and its effect on wound healing Songklanakarin
J Sci Technol, 28 (5) (2006), pp. 897–910
Chan E, Elevitch CR. Species profiles for Pacific island agroforestry, 2006. [Online]. Available from: www.traditionaltree.org [Accessed on November 03, 2010].

NMCE. Report on copra. National Multi-commodity Exchange of India Limited; 2007, 1-14.

Dayrit CS. The truth about coconut oil: The drugstore in a bottle. Philippines: Anvil Publishing, Inc; 2005.

Vestlund L. The healing power of organic virgin coconut oil, 2009. [Online]. Available from: http://cocofat.com/virgin-coconut-oilvcor.html

United States Department of Agriculture (USDA). National nutrient database for standard reference, Nuts, coconut water, 2008.
[Online]. Available from: http://www.nal.usda.gov/fnic/foodcomp/cgi-bin/list_nut_edit.pl/. [Accessed on December 8, 2009].
Yong WJWH, Ge L, Ng YF, Tan SN. The chemical composition and biological properties of coconut (Cocos nucifera L.). Molecules
2009; 14: 5144-5164.

Bawalan DD, Chapman KR. Virgin coconut oil: Production manual for micro-and village-scale processing. FAO Regional Office for Asia and the Pacific, Bangkok: Food and Agriculture Organization of the United Nations; 2006, p. 1-112.

Marina AM, Che Man YB, Nazimah SAH, Amin I. Chemical properties of virgin coconut oil. J Am Oil Chem Soc 2009; 86: 301-307.
Effiong GS, Ebong PE, Eyong EU, Uwah AJ, Ekong UE. Amelioration of chloramphenicol induced toxicity in rats by coconut water. J Appl Sc Res 2010; 6(4): 331-335.

Loki AL, Rajamohan T. Hepatoprotective and antioxidant effect of tender coconut water on CCl4 induced liver injury in rats. Indian J Biochem Biophy 2003; 40: 354-357.
Bankar GR, Nayak PG, Bansal P, Paul P, Pai KSR, Singla RK, et al. Vasorelaxant and antihypertensive effect of Cocos nucifera Linn. endocarp on isolated rat thoracic aorta and DOCA salt induced hypertensive rats. J Ethnopharmacol 2010. doi:10.1016/j.jep.2010.11.047.

Manisha DebMandal et al./Asian Pacific Journal of Tropical Medicine (2011)241-247 247
Nevin KG, Rajamohan T. Virgin coconut oil supplemented diet increases the antioxidant status in rats. Food Chem 2005; 99: 260-266.

Enig MG. Coconut: In support of good health in the 21st Century, 2004. [Online]. Available from: http://www.apcc.org.sg/special. htm. [Accessed on December 27, 2010].

Nevin KG, Rajamohan T. Beneficial effects of virgin coconut oil on lipid parameters and in vitro LDL oxidation. Clin Biochem 2004; 37: 830-835.

Nevin KG, Rajamohan T. Influence of virgin coconut oil on blood coagulation factors, lipid levels and LDL oxidation in cholesterol fed Sprague-Dawley rats. Eur e-J Clin Nutr Metabol 2007; e1-e8.

Müller H, Lindman AS, Blomfeldt A, Seljeflot I, Pedersen JI. A diet rich in coconut oil reduces diurnal postprandial variations in circulating tissue plasminogen activator antigen and fasting lipoprotein(a) compared with a diet rich in unsaturated fat in women. J Nutr 2003; 133(11): 3422-3427.

Ibrahim AI, Obeid MT, Jouma MJ, Moasis GA, Al-Richane WL, Kindermann I, et al. Detection of herpes simplex virus, cytomegalovirus and Epstein-Barr virus DNA in atherosclerotic plaques and in unaffected bypass grafts. J Clin Virol 2005; 32(1): 29-32.

Esquenazi D, Wigg MD, Miranda MM, Rodrigues HM, Tostes JB, Rozental S, et al. Antimicrobial and antiviral activities of polyphenolics from Cocos nucifera Linn. (Palmae) husk fiber extract. Res Microbiol 2002; 153(10):647-652.

Mini S, Rajamohan T. Influence of coconut kernel protein on lipid metabolism in alcohol fed rats. Indian J Exp Biol 2004; 42(1): 53-57.

Eckarstein V, Noter JR, Assmann G. High density lipoproteins and atherosclerosis. Role of cholesterol efflux and reverse cholesterol transport. Arterioscler Thromb Vasc Biol 2002; 21: 13-27.

Abate MA, Moore TL. Monooctanoin use for gallstone dissolution. Drug Intell Clin Pharm 1985; 19: 708-713.

Daftary GV, Pai SA, Shanbhag GN. Stable emulsion compositions for intravenous administration having preservatie efficacy. United States Patent Application 20080262084. (10/23/2008).

Oyi AR, Onaolapo JA, Obi RC. Formulation and antimicrobial studies of coconut (Cocos nucifera Linne) Oil. Res J Appl S Eng Tech 2010; 2(2): 133-137.

Thormar H, Hilmarsson H, Bergsson G. Stable concentrated emulsions of the 1-monoglyceride of capric acid (monocaprin) with microbicidal activities against the food-borne bacteria Campylobacter jejuni, Salmonella spp., and Escherichia coli. Appl Environ Microbiol 2006; 72(1): 522-526.
Thormar H, Hilmarsson H. The role of microbicidal lipids in host defense against pathogens and their potential as therapeutic agents. Chem Phy lipids 2007; 150(1): 1-11.

Mandal S, Mandal MD, Pal NK, Saha K. Synergistic antiStaphylococcus aureus activity of amoxicillin in combination with Emblica officinalis and Nymphae odorata extracts. Asian Pacific J Trop Med 2010; 3: 711-714.

Mandal S, Mandal M, Pal NK. Antibacterial potential of Azadirachta indica seed and Bacopa monniera leaf extracts against multidrug resistant Salmonella enterica serovar Typhi isolates.
Archives Med Sci 2007; 3: 14-18.

Obi RC, Oyi AR, Onaolapo JA. Antimicrobial activities of coconut (Cocos nucifera Linne) oil. 2nd Annual National Scientific Conference. Ahmadu Bello University, Zaria, Nigeria: National Association of Pharmacists in Academia; 2005, p. 81.
Alviano DS, Rodrigues KF, Leitão SG, Rodrigues ML, Matheus ML, Fernández PD, et al.

Antinociceptive and free radical scavenging activities of Cocos nucifera L. (Palmae) husk fiber aqueous extract. J Ethnopharmacol 2004; 92: 269-273. Alviano WS, Alviano DS, Diniz CG, Antoniolli AR, Alviano
CS, Farias LM, et al.

In vitro antioxidant potential of medicinal plant extracts and their activities against oral bacteria based on Brazilian folk medicine. Arch Oral Biol 2008; 53: 545-552.
Taheri JB, Espineli FW, Lu H, Asayesh M, Bakshi M, Nakhostin MR.

Antimicrobial effect of coconut flour on oral microflora: An in vitro study. Res J Biol Scs 2010; 5(6): 456-459.

Barnabé W, de Mendonça Neto T, Pimenta FC, Pegoraro LF, Scolaro JM.

Efficacy of sodium hypochlorite and coconut soap used as disinfecting agents in the reduction of denture stomatitis, Streptococcus mutans and Candida albicans. J Oral Rehabil 2004; 31(5): 453-459.

Agero AL, Verallo-Rowell VM. A randomized double-blind controlled trial comparing extra virgin coconut oil with mineral oil as a moisturizer for mild to moderate xerosis. Dermatitis 2004; 15:109-116.

Carpo BG, Verallo-Rowell VM, Kabara JJ. Novel antibacterial activity of monolaurin compared with conventional antibiotics against organisms from skin infections: an in vitro study. Drugs Dermatol 2007; 6(10): 991-998.

Verallo-Rowell VM, Dillague KM, Syah-Tjundawan BS. Novel antibacterial and emollient effects of coconut and virgin olive oils in adult atopic dermatitis. Dermatitis 2008; 19(6): 308-315.
Arora R, Chawla R, Marwah R, Arora P, Sharma RK, Kaushik V, et al.

Potential of complementary and alternative medicine in preventive management of novel H1N1 flu (Swine flu) pandemic: thwarting potential disasters in the Bud. Evid-Based Complement Alternat Med 2011. doi:10.1155/2011/586506.

Rihakova Z, Filip V, Plockova M, Smidrkal J, Cervenkova R. Inhibition of Aspergillus niger DMF 0801 by monoacylglycerols prepared from coconut oil. Czech J Food Sci 2002; 20: 48-52.

Ogbolu DO, Oni AA, Daini OA, Oloko AP. In vitro antimicrobial properties of coconut oil on Candida sp. in Ibadan, Nigeria. J Med Food 2007; 10(2): 384-387.

Mendonca-Filho RR, Rodrigues IA, Alviano DS, Santos ALS, Soares RMA, Alviano CS, et al. Leishmanicidal activity of polyphenolic-rich extract from husk fiber of Cocos nucifera Linn. (Palmae). Res Microbiol 2004; 155: 136-143.

Sosnowska J, Balslev H. American palm ethnomedicine: A metaanalysis.
J Ethnobiol Ethnomed 2009; 5: 43.

Koschek PR, Alviano DS, Alviano CS, Gattas CR. The husk fiber of Cocos nucifera L. (Palmae) is a source of anti-neoplastic activity. Braz J Med Biol Res 2007; 40: 1339-1343.

Winarsi H, Hernayanti, Purwanto A. Virgin coconut oil (VCO) enriched with Zn as immunostimulator for vaginal Candidiasis patient. Hayati J Biosc 2008; 15(4): 135-139.

Vigila AG, Baskaran X. Immunomodulatory effect of coconut protein on cyclophosphamide induced immune suppressed Swiss Albino mice. Ethnobot Leaflets 2008; 12: 1206-1212.

Salil G, Nevin KG, Rajamohan T. Arginine rich coconut kernel protein modulates diabetes in alloxan treated rats. Chemico-Biol Interact 2010. doi:10.1016/j.cbi.2010.10.015.

Kneiflova J, Slosarek M, Melichercikova V, Paríkova J. Microbicidal effect of Lautercide, a new disinfectant. Cesk Epidemiol Mikrobiol Imunol 1992; 41(6): 355-361.

Dautel H, Hilker M, Kahl O, Siems K. Verwendung von Dodecansäureals Zeckenrepellent. Patentschrift DE 199 25 838 C
1. Deutsches Patent- und Markenamt. (01.03.2001).
2.
Sylla M, Konan L, Doannio JM, Traore S. Evaluation of the efficacity of coconut (Cocos nucifera), palm nut (Eleais guineensis) and gobi (Carapa procera) lotions and creams in

individual protection against Simulium damnosum s.l. bites in Cote d'Ivoire.
Bull Soc Pathol Exot 2003; 96(2):104-109.

Robeerto CA. Cocobiodiesel. Coconut methyl ester (CME) as petrodiesel quality enhancer. Dept. Agr. Philippine Coconut Authority; 2001, p.1-37.

Radenahmad N, Vongvatcharanon U, Withyachumnarnkul B, Connor JR. Serum levels of 17β-estradiol in ovariectomized rats fed young-coconut-juice and its effect on wound healing
Songklanakarin J Sci Technol 2006; 28(5): 897-910.

Cordyceps sinensis

Life Sciences
Volume 60, Issue 25, 16 May 1997, Pages 2349–2359
Effect of Cordyceps sinensis on the proliferation and differentiation of human leukemic U937 cells
Yu-Jen Chen1, 3, *, Ming-Shi Shiao1, 2, Shiuh-Sheng Lee4, Sheng-Yuan Wang, 1,

Life Sciences
Volume 60, Issue 25, 16 May 1997, Pages 2349–2359
Effect of Cordyceps sinensis on the proliferation and differentiation of human leukemic U937 cells
Yu-Jen Chen1, 3, *, Ming-Shi Shiao1, 2, Shiuh-Sheng Lee4, Sheng-Yuan Wang,

The American Journal of Chinese Medicine
An International Journal of Comparative Medicine East and West
Volume 24, Issue 02, 1996
Yuh-Chi Kuo et al, Am. J. Chin. Med. 24, 111 (1996). DOI: 10.1142/S0192415X96000165
Cordyceps sinensis as an Immunomodulatory Agent

Cancer Investigation
Volume 12, Issue 6, 1994

Growth Inhibitors Against Tumor Cells in Cordyceps sinensis Other than Cordycepin and Polysaccharides
Growth Inhibitors Against Tumor Cells in Cordyceps sinensis Other than Cordycepin and Polysaccharides
DOI:10.3109/07357909409023046

Yuh-Chi Kuoa*, Ching-Yuang Linb, Wei-Jern Tsaia, Chia-Ling Wua, Chieh-Fu Chena & Ming-Shi Shiaoc
pages 611-615

Bioscience, Biotechnology, and Biochemistry
Volume 66, Issue 2, 2002
Activation of Macrophages and the Intestinal Immune System by an Orally Administered Decoction from Cultured Mycelia of Cordyceps sinensis

Activation of Macrophages and the Intestinal Immune System by an Orally Administered Decoction from Cultured Mycelia of Cordyceps sinensis
DOI:10.1271/bbb.66.407
Jong-Ho KOHae, Kwang-Won YUb, Hyung-Joo SUHc, Yang-Moon CHOId & Tae-Seok AHNa
pages 407-411

Biological and Pharmaceutical Bulletin
Vol. 26 (2003) No. 5 P 691-694
http://doi.org/10.1248/bpb.26.691
Antifatigue and Antistress Effect of the Hot-Water Fraction from Mycelia of Cordyceps sinensis
Jong-Ho Koh1), Kyung-Mi Kim1), Jin-Man Kim2), Jae-Chul Song3), Hyung-Joo Suh2)

Journal of Ethnopharmacology
Volume 114, Issue 1, 8 October 2007, Pages 78–85
Evaluation of the anti-inflammatory and anti-proliferation tumoral cells activities of Antrodia camphorata, Cordyceps sinensis, and Cinnamomum osmophloeum bark extracts
Yerra Koteswara Raoa, Shih-Hua Fangb, Yew-Min Tzenga,

'CSE improved the activity of superoxide dismutase, glutathione peroxidase and catalase and lowered the level of lipid peroxidation and monoamine oxidase activity in the aged mice. The study demonstrated that CSE can improve the brain function and antioxidative enzyme activity in mice with d-galactose-induced senescence and promote sexual function in castrated rats. All of these findings suggest that CSE has an antiaging effect'.
Antiaging effect of Cordyceps sinensis extract
Deng-Bo Ji1, Jia Ye1,*, Chang-Ling Li1, Yu-Hua Wang1, Jiong Zhao1 andShao-Qing Cai2

L-Carnitine

Current Medical Research and Opinion
Volume 11, Issue 10, 1990
Double-blind, placebo controlled study of acetyl-l-carnitine in patients with Alzheimer's dementia
DOI:10.1185/03007999009112690
G. Rai[a], G. Wright[a], L. Scott[a], B. Beston[a], J. Rest[a] & A. N. Exton-Smith[a]
pages 638-647

This meta-analysis showed very good results with L-Carnitine:
International Clinical Psychopharmacology:
March 2003 - Volume 18 - Issue 2 - pp 61-71
Meta-analysis of double blind randomized controlled clinical trials of acetyl-L-carnitine versus placebo in the treatment of mild cognitive impairment and mild Alzheimer's disease
Montgomery, Stuart A.[a]; Thal, L.J.[b]; Amrein, R.[c]

This long term study also showed good results:
Long-term acetyl-L-carnitine treatment in Alzheimer's disease
A. Spagnoli, MD, U. Lucca, PhD, G. Menasce, MD, L. Bandera, MD, G. Cizza, MD, G. Forloni, PhD, M. Tettamanti, PhD, L. Frattura, MD, P. Tiraboschi, MD, M. Comelli, PhD, U. Senin, MD, A. Longo, MD, A. Petrini, MD, G. Brambilla, MD, A. Belloni, PhD, C. Negri, MD, F. Cavazzuti, MD, A. Salsi, MD, P. Calogero, MD, E. Parma, MD, M. Stramba-Badiale, MD, S. Vitali, MD, G. Andreoni, MD, M. R. Inzoli, MD, G. Santus, MD, R. Caregnato, MD, M. Peruzza, MD, M. Favaretto, MD, C. Bozeglav, PhD, M. Alberoni,

MD, D. De Leo, MD, L. Serraiotto, MD, A. Baiocchi, MD, S. Scoccia, MD, P. Culotta, MD and D. Ieracitano, MD

doi: http://dx.doi.org/10.1212/WNL.41.11.1726 Neurology November 1991 vol. 41 no. 11 1726

Epilepsia Official Journal of the International League Against Epilepsy
l-Carnitine Supplementation in Childhood Epilepsy: Current Perspectives

Darryl C. De Vivo[1,*], Timothy P. Bohan[2], David L. Coulter[3], Fritz E. Dreifuss[4], Robert S. Greenwood[5], Douglas R. Nordli Jr.[1], W. Donald Shields[6], Carl E. Stafstrom[7] and Ingrid Tein[8]
Article first published online: 3 AUG 2005
DOI: 10.1111/j.1528-1157.1998.tb01315.x

l-Carnitine l-tartrate supplementation favorably affects markers of recovery from exercise stress
Jeff S. Volek, William J. Kraemer, Martyn R. Rubin, Ana L. Gómez, Nicholas A. Ratamess, Paula Gaynor
American Journal of Physiology - Endocrinology and Metabolism
Published 1 February 2002 **Vol.** 282 **no.** 2, E474-E482 **DOI:** 10.1152/ajpendo.00277.2001

Nutrition Volume 20, Issues 7–8, July–August 2004, Pages 709–715 Supplementation of l-carnitine in athletes: does it make sense? ☆ Heidrun Karlic, PhD[a], Alfred Lohninger, PhD[b]

Mayo Clinic Proceedings
Volume 88, Issue 6, June 2013, Pages 544–551
L-Carnitine in the Secondary Prevention of Cardiovascular Disease: Systematic Review and Meta-analysis
James J. DiNicolantonio, PharmD[a,*], Carl J. Lavie, MD[b,c], Hassan Fares, MD[b], Arthur R. Menezes, MD[b], James H. O'Keefe, MD[d]

Probiotics

Probiotics: Considerations for Human Health
Mary Ellen Sanders Ph D
DOI: http://dx.doi.org/10.1301/nr.2003.marr.91-99 91-99 First published online: 1 March 2003
Medical References- Chlorophyll, Cereal Grasses

GENERAL ARTICLES CURRENT SCIENCE, VOL. 88, NO. 11, 10 JUNE 20051745 1.Metchinkoff, E., The Prolongation of Life, Putmans Sons, New York, 1908, pp. 151–183.2.Pollman, D. S., Danielson, D. M. and Peo Jr. E. R.,

Effects of micro-bial feed additives on performance of starter and growing-finishing pigs. J. Anim. Sci., 1980, 51, 577–581.3.Garvie, E. L., Cole, C. B., Fuller, R. and Hewitt, D.,

The effect of yoghurt on some components of the gut microflora and the meta-bolism of lactose in the rat. J. Appl. Bacteriol., 1984, 56, 237–245.4.Gilliland, S. E., Nelson, C. R. and Maxwell, C.,

Assimilation of cholesterol by Lactobacillus acidophilus. Appl. Environ. Micro-biol., 1985, 49, 377–381.5.Manisha, N., Ashar and Prajapati, J. B.,

Role of probiotic cultures and fermented milks in combating blood cholesterol. Indian J. Micro-biol., 2001, 41, 75–86.6.Rettiger, L. F. and Chaplin, H. A.,

A treatise on the transformation of the intestinal flora with special reference to the implantation of Bacillus acidophilus, Yale University Press, Connecticut, 1921.7.Reddy, G. V., Shahini, K. M. and Banerjee, M. R.,

Inhibitory effect of the yoghurt on Ehrlich ascites tumour cell proliferation. J. Natl. Cancer Res. Inst., 1993, 50, 815–817.8.Rowland, I. R. and Grasso, P., Degradation of N-nitrosamine by intestinal bacteria. Appl. Microbiol., 1975, 29, 7–12.9.Fuller, R.,

Probiotics in man and animals. J. Appl. Bacteriol., 1989, 66, 365–378.10.Colombel, J. F., Cartot, A., Neut, C. and Romond, C.,

Yogurt with Bifidobacterium longum reduces erythromycin-induced gastroin-testinal effects. Lancet, 1987, 11, 43.11.Thronton, G. M.,

Probiotic bacteria selection of Lactobacillus and Bifidobacterium strains from the healthy human gastrointestinal tract, characterization of a novel Lactobacillus-derived antibacte-rial protein (thesis), National Univ., Ireland, 1996.12.Gilliland, S. E. and Speck, M. L.,

Deconjugaton of bile acids by intestinal lactobacilli. Appl. Environ. Microbiol., 1977, 33, 15–18.13.Harrison, V. C. and Peat, G., Serum cholesterol and bowel flora in the new born. Am. J. Clin. Nutr., 1975, 28, 1351–1355.14.Grunewald, K. K.,

Serum cholesterol levels in rats fed with skim milk fermented by Lactobacillus acidophilus. J. Food Sci., 1982, 47, 2078–2079.15.Lin, S. Y., Ayres, J. W., Winkler, W. and Sandine, W. E.,

Lacto-bacillus effects on cholesterol: in vitroandin vivo results. J. Dairy Sci.,1989, 72, 2885–2899.16.De Roos, N. M., Schouten, G. and Katan, M. B.,

Yoghurt enriched with Lactobacillus acidophilus does not lower blood lipids in healthy men and women with normal to borderline high serum cholesterol levels. Eur. J. Clin. Nutr., 1999, 53, 277–280.17.Tahri, K., Grill, J. P. and Schneider, F.,

Bifidobacteria strain behaviour toward cholesterol: Coprecipitation with bile salts and assimilation.Curr. Microbiol., 1996, 33, 187–193.18.Lin, S. Y. and Chen, C. T., Reduction of cholesterol by Lactobacillusacidophilus in culture broth. J. Food Drug Anal., 2000, 8, 97–102.19.Mitsuoka, T.,

Intestinal flora and cancer. In Second Annual Natio-nal Symposium for Lactic Acid Bacteria and Health, Korea, 1981, pp. 16–40. 20. Hirayana, T.,

An epidemiological study on the effect of diet, especially of milk on the incidence of stomach cancer. In Abstr. IX, In-ternational Cancer Congress, Tokyo, 1966, p. 713. 21. Yano, K.,

Effect of vegetable juices and milk on alkylating activity of N-methyl-N-nitrosourea. J. Agric. Food Chem., 1979, 27, 456–458. 22. Gaskill, S. P., McGuire, W. L., Osborne, C. K. and Stern, M. P.,

Breast cancer mortality and diet in the United States. Cancer Res., 1979, 39, 3628–3637. 23. Friend, B. A. and Sahani, K. M., Antitumour properties of lacto-bacilli. J. Food Prot., 1984, 47, 717–723. 24. Pool-Zobel, B. L. et al.,

Lactobacillus and Bifidobacterium medi-ated antigenotoxicity in the colon of rats. Nutr. Cancer, 1996, 29, 365–380. 25. Rowland, I. R., Rumney, C. J., Coutts, J. T. and Lievense, L. C.,

Effect of Bifidobacteriumlongum on gut bacterial metabolism and carcinogen-induced aberrant crypt foci in rats. Carcinogenesis, 1998, 19, 281–285. 26. McIntosh, G. H., Royle, P. J. and Playne, M. J.,

A probiotic strain of L. acidophilus reduces DMH-induced large intestinal tumors in male Sprague–Dawley rats. Nutr. Cancer, 1999, 35, 153–159. 27. Friend, B. A. and Sahani, K. M., Antitumour properties of Lacto-bacilli and dairy products fermented by lactobacilli. J. Food Prot., 1984, 47, 717–723. 28. Aso, Y. and Akazan, H.,

Prophylactic effect of a Lactobacillus caseipreparation on the recurrence of superficial bladder cancer. Urol. Int., 1992, 49, 125–129. 29. Reddy, B. S. and Rivenson, A.,

Inhibitory effect of Bifidobacte-rium longum colon, mammary and liver carcinogenesis induced by 2-amino, 3-methylimidazo (4,5-f-quinoline), a food mutagen. Can-cer Res., 1993, 53, 3914–

30. Oberreuther-Moschner, D. L., Jahreis, G., Rechkemner, G. and PoolZobel, B. L.,

Dietary intervention with the probiotics Lactobacil-lus acidophilus 145 and Bifidobacterium longum 913 modulates the potential of human faecal water to induce damage in HT29 clone 19A cells. Br. J. Nutr., 2004, 91, 925–932.

31. Burns, A. J. and Rowland, I. R.,

Anticarcinogenicity of probiotics and prebiotics. Curr. Issues Intest. Microbiol., 2000, 2, 13–24.

32. Pelletier, X., Laure-Boussuge, S. and Donazzolo, Y.,

Hydrogen excretion upon ingestion of dairy products in lactose intolerant male subjects: Importance of the live flora. Eur. J. Clin. Nutr.,2001, 55, 509–512.

33. Birge, S. J., Kautmann, H. T., Cuatrecasaa, P. and Whedon, G. D.,

Osteoporosis, intestinal lactose deficiency and low dietary calcium intake. N. Engl. J. Med., 1967, 276, 445.

34. Kalliomaki, M., Salminen, S., Arvilommi, H., Kero, P., Koskinen, P. and Isolauri, E.,

Probiotics in primary prevention of atopic dis-ease: A randomized placebo-controlled trial. Lancet, 2001, 357, 1076–1079.

35. Rautava, S., Kalliomaki, M. and Isolauri, E.,

Probiotics during pregnancy and breast-feeding might confer immunomodulatory protection against atopic disease in the infant. J. Allergy Clin. Im-munol.,2002, 109, 119–121.

36. Majamaa, H. and Isolauri, E.,

Probiotics: A novel approach in the management of food allergy. J. Allergy Clin. Immunol., 1997, 99, 179–185.

37. Pathmakanthan, S., Meance, S. and Edwards, C. A.,

Probiotics: A review of human studies to date and methodological approaches. Microb. Ecol. Health Dis., 2000, 2, 10–30.

38. Majamaa, H., Isolauri, E., Saxelin, M. and Vesikari, T.,

Lactic acid bacteria in the treatment of acute rotavirus gastroenteritis. J. Pediatr. Gastroenterol. Nutr., 1995, 20, 333–338.39.Pedone, C. A., Bernabeu, A. O., Postaire, E. R., Bouley, C. F. and Reinert, P.,

The effect of supplementation with milk fermented by Lactobacillus casei (strain DN-114 001) on acute diarrhoea in children attending day-care centres. Int. J. Clin. Pract.,1999, 53, 179–184.40.Saavedra, J. M., Bauman, N. A., Oung, I., Perman, J. A. and Yolken, R. H.,

Feeding of Bifidobacterium bifidum and Strepto-coccus thermophilus to infants in hospital for prevention of diar-rhoea and shedding of rotavirus. Lancet, 1994, 344, 1046–1049.41.D'Souza, A. L., Rajkumar, C., Cooke, J. and Bulpitt, C. J.,

Probiotics in prevention of antibiotic associated diarrhoea: meta-analysis. Br. Med. J., 2002, 324, 1361–1366.42. Gionchetti, P., Rizzello, F. and Venturi, A.,

Oral bacteriotherapy as maintenance treatment in patients with chronic pouchitis: A double blind placebo controlled trial. Gastroenterology, 2000, 119, 305–309.Received 6 November 2004; revised accepted 27 January 2005

Menopause. 2006 Nov-Dec;13(6):862-77; quiz 878-80.
The role of calcium in peri- and postmenopausal women: 2006 position statement of the North American Menopause Society.
Milk, Milk Products, and Disease Free Health: An Updated Overview

Critical Reviews in Food Science and Nutrition
Volume 52, Issue 4, 2012:10.1080/10408398.2010.500231
R. Nagpala, P. V. Behareb, M. Kumarb, D. Mohaniac, M. Yadavd, S. Jaine, S. Menonf, O. Parkashg, F. Marottah, E. Minellih, C. J.K. Henryi & H. Yadavj
pages 321-333

Wheatgrass

Hughes and Letner. "Chlorophyll and Hemoglobin Regeneration," <u>American Journal of Medical Science</u>, 188, 206 (1936)

Patek. "Chlorophyll and Regeneration of Blood," <u>Archives of Internal Medicine.</u> 57, 76 (1936)

Kohler, Elvahjem and Hart. "Growth Stimulating Properties of Grass Juice," <u>Science</u>. 83, 445 (1936)

Kohler, Elvahjem and Hart. "The Relation of the Grass Juice Factor to Guinea Pig Nutrition." <u>Journal of Nutrition,</u> 15, 445 (1938)

Rhoads. "The Relation of Vitamin K to the Hemorrhagic Tendency in Obstructive Jaundice (Dehydrated Cereal Grass as the Source of Vitamin K). <u>Journal of Medicine,</u> 112, 2259, (1939)

Waddall. "Effect of Vitamin K on the Clotting Time of the Prothrombin and the Blood (Dehydrated Cereal Grass as the Source of Vitamin K)." Journal of Medicine. 112, 2259 (1939)

Illingworth. "Hemmorrhage in Jaundice (Use of Dehydrated Cereal Grass)." <u>Lancet.</u> 236. 1031 (1939)

Kohler, Randle and Wagner. "The Grass Juice Factor." <u>Journal of Biological Chemistry.</u> 128, 1w (1939)

Friedman and Friedman. "Gonadotropic Extracts from Green Leaves." <u>American Journal of Physiology.</u> 125, 486, (1939)

Randle, Sober and Kohler. "The Distribution of the Grass Juice Factor in Plant and Animal Materials." <u>The Journal of Nutrition.</u> 20, 459 (1940)

Gomez, Hartman and Dryden. "Influence of Oat Juice Extract Upon the Age of Sexual Maturity in Rats. <u>The Journal of Dairy Science.</u> 24, 507 (1941)

Miller. "Chlorophyll for Healing." Science News Letter. March 15, 171 (1941)

Gomez. "Further Evidence of the Existence and Specificiey of an Orally Active Sex Maturity Factor (s) in Plant Juice Preparations." The Journal of Dairy Science. 25, 705 (1942)

Kohler. "The Effect of Stage of Growth on the Chemistry of the Grasses." The Journal of Biological Chemistry. 215-23 (1944)

Boehme. "The Treatment of Chronic Leg Ulcers with Special Reference to Ointment Containing Water Soluble Chlorophyll." Cahey Clinical Bulletin. 4, 242 (1946)

Bowers. "Chlorophyll in Wound Healing and Suppurative Disease." The American Journal of Surgery. 71, 37 (1947)

Colio and Babb. "Study of a New Stimulatory Growth Factor," Journal of Biological Chemistry, 174, 405 (1948)

Juul-Moller and Middelsen. "Treatment of Intestinal Disease with Solutions of Water Soluble Chlorophyll." The Review of Gastroenterology. 15, 549 (1948)

Carpenter. "Clinical Experiences with Chlorophyll Preparations with Particular Reference to Chronic Osteomyelitis and Chronic Ulcer." American Journal of Surgery. 77, 267 (1949)

Offenkrantz. "Water-Soluble Chlorophyll in Ulcers of Long Duration." Review of Gastroenterology, 17, 359-67 (1950)

Anselmi. "Clinical Use of Chlorophyll and Derivatives." (??H or M) Minerva Medica. 2, 1313-14 (1950)
Lam and Brush. "Chlorophyll and Wound Healing: Experimental and Clinical Sudy," American Journal of Surgery. 80, 204-20 (1950)

Granick. "Structural and Functional Relationships between Heme and Chlorophyll." The Harvey Lectures. (1943-1949)

Cheney. "Antipeptic Ulcer Dietary Factor." The Journal of the American Dietetic Association. 26, 668 (1950)

Cheney. "The Nature of the Antipeptic Ulcer Factor." Stanford Medical Bulletin, 8, 144 (1950)

Sonsky. "Vitamin K Influence of Preventative Prenatal Administration," Ceskolovenska Gyneakologia, 29, 197 (1950)

Mossberg. "Vitamin K Treatment of Acute Hepatitus." British Medical Journal. 1, 1382-84 (1961)

Reid. "Treatment of Hypoprothrombinemia with Orally Administered Vitamin K." Quarterly Bulletin: Northwestern University Medical School. 25. 292-95 (1951)

Dohan, Richardson, Stribley and Gyorgy. "The Estrogenic Effects of Extracts of Spring Rye Grass." Journal of the American Veterinary Medicine Association. 118, 323 (1951)

Kohler and Graham. "A Chick Growth Factor Found in Leafy Green Vegetation," Poultry Science. 30, 484 ((1951)

Paloscia and Pallotta. "Chlorophyll in Therapy." Lotta Controlla Tubercolosi, 22, 738-40 (1952)

Shattan and Kutcher. "Effect of Chlorophyll on Postextraction Healing." Journal of Oral Surgery. 46, 324 (1952)

Kutcher and Chilton. "Clinical Use of Chlorophyll Dentifrice." Journal of the American Dental Association. 46, 420-22 (1953)

Kohler. "The Unidentified Vitamins of Grass and Alfalfa." Feedstuffs Magazine. August 8 (1953).

Dunham. "Differential Inhibition of Virus Hemagglutination by Clorophyllin." Proceedings of the Society for Experimental Biology and Medicine. 87, 431-33 (1954)

Gandolfi. "Repitelizing Potency Exerted on Cornea by Chlorophyll." <u>Annali de Ottalmologiale Clinica Oculistica.</u> 80, 131-42 (1954)

Borelli. "Chlorophyll (for Acne Therapy). Der Hautarzt. 6, 120-24 (1955)

Gandolfo. "Antismotic Activity of Chlorophyllin." <u>Rendiconti Instituto Superiore de Sanita.</u> 18, 641-48 (1955)

Offenkrantz. "Complete Healing (Peptic Ulcer) with Water-Soluble Chlorophyll." <u>American Journal of Gastroenterology.</u> 24, 182-85 (1955)

Wennig. Modification and Inhibition of Resorption of Urinary Substances with Chlorophyllin," <u>Wiener Medizinishe Wochenschrift.</u> 105, 885-87 (1955)

Ammon and Wolfe. "Does Chloro;hyll have Bactericidal and Bacteriostatic Activity?" <u>Arzneimettel-Forschung.</u> 5, 312-14 (1955)

Bertram and Weinstock. "A Clinical Evaluation of Chlorophyll, Benzocain and Urea Ointment in Treatment of Minor Infections of the Foot." Journal of the American Podiatry Association. 19, 366 (1959)

The Scandanavian Journal of Gastroenterology, Volume 37, Number 4/April 1, 2002, pages 444-449 talks of a study titled: "Wheat Grass Juice in the Treatment of Active Distal Ulcerative Colitis: A Randomized Double-blind Placebo-controlled Trial." Conclusion: "Wheat grass juice appeared effective and safe as a single or adjuvant treatment of distal UC."References
Journal of Nutrition; Tart Cherry Juice Decreases Oxidative Stress in Healthy Older Men and Women; T Traustadóttir, SS Davies, AA Stock, et al.; Aug 2009

Functional Foods in Health and Disease
Vol 1, No 11 (2011) > Rana
Living life the natural way – Wheatgrass and Health
Satyavati Rana, Jaspreet Kaur Kamboj, Vandana Gandhi

Shiitake Mushroom

Advances in Applied Microbiology 1993
by Academic Press

Journal of the American Academy of Dermatology
Volume 24, Issue 1, January 1991, Pages 64-66
Allergy and toxicodermia from shiitake mushrooms
Kyllikki Tarvainen, MD *, 1, Jukka-Pekka Salonen, MD 1, Lasse Kanerva, MD, PhD 1, Tuula Estlander, MD 1, Helena Keskinen, MD 1, Tapio Rantanen, MD

Chemical and Pharmaceutical Bulletin
Vol. 35 (1987) No. 6 P 2459-2464
http://doi.org/10.1248/cpb.35.2459
Antitumor Mechanisms of Orally Administered Shiitake Fruit Bodies
HIROAKI NANBA, HISATORA KURODA1)

Vol. 34, No. 1, 2000
Issue release date: January–February 2000
Caries Res 2000;34:94–98
(DOI:10.1159/000016559)
Anticaries Effect of a Component from Shiitake (an Edible Mushroom)
Shouji N. · Takada K. · Fukushima K. · Hirasawa M.

Chemical and Pharmaceutical Bulletin
Vol. 35 (1987) No. 6 P 2453-2458
http://doi.org/10.1248/cpb.35.2453
Antitumor Action of Shiitake (Lentinus edodes) Fruit Bodies Orally Administered to Mice
HIROAKI NANBA1), KANICHI MORI2), TETSURO TOYOMASU2), HISATORA KURODA1)

H. Nanba, K. Mori, T. Toyomasu and H. Kuroda, Chem. Pharm. Bull., 35, 2453 (1987).

Y. Y. Maeda, G. Chihara and K. Ishimura, Nature (London), 52,250 (1974).

J. Hamuro, H. Wagner and M. Röllinghoff, Cell Immunol., 38,328 (1978).

M. Ito, H. Suzuki, N. Nakano, N. Yamashita, E. Sugiyama, M. Maruyama, K. Hoshino and S. Yano, Gann, 74,128 (1983).

O. H. Lowry, N. J. Rosebrough, A. L. Farr and R. J. Randall, J. Biol. Chem., 193,265 (1951).

K. Hashimoto and T. Kitagawa, Cell Antigen, IV, 352 (1972).

N. Saijo, A. Ozaki, Y. Beppu, N. Irimajiri, M. Shibuya, E. Shimizu, T. Takizawa, T. Taniguchi and A. Hoshi, Gann, 74,137 (1983).

H. Nakajima, S. Abe, Y. Masuko, J. Tsubouchi, M. Yamazaki and D. Mizuno, Gann, 72,723 (1981).

J. Hamuro, H. Wagner and M. Röllinghoff, Cell Immunol., 38,328 (1978).

J. Hamuro, M. Rollinghoff and H. Wagner,.Cancer Res., 38, 3080 (1978).

Sour Cherries

Journal of Agriculture and Food Chemistry; Oxidation of Cholesterol and beta-Sitosterol and Prevention by Natural Antioxidants; G Xu, L Guan, J Sun and ZY Chen; Sep 2009

British Journal of Sports Medicine; Efficacy of a tart cherry juice blend in preventing the symptoms of muscle damage; DA Connolly, MP McHugh, OL Padilla-Zakour, et al.; Dec 2006

USDA National Nutrient Database: Cherries, Sour European
Review for Medical and Pharmacological Science: Quercetin potentially attenuates cadmium induced oxidative stress mediated cardiotoxicity and dyslipidemia in rats " Study: Tart Cherry Juice Increases Sleep Time In Adults With Insomnia "University of Marlyland Medical Center: Quercetin
American Institute of Cancer Research: Foods That Fight Cancer

Spirulina

Clin Toxicol (Phila). 2006;44(2):135-41.
Efficacy of spirulina extract plus zinc in patients of chronic arsenic poisoning: a randomized placebo-controlled study.
Misbahuddin M1, Islam AZ, Khandker S, Ifthaker-Al-Mahmud, Islam N, Anjumanara.

Environ Toxicol Pharmacol. 2012 Nov;34(3):721-6. doi: 10.1016/j.etap.2012.09.016. Epub 2012 Oct 8.
Preventive effect of phycocyanin from Spirulina platensis on alloxan-injured mice.
Ou Y1, Lin L, Pan Q, Yang X, Cheng X.

Pharm Biol. 2013 May;51(5):539-44. doi: 10.3109/13880209.2012.747545. Epub 2013 Feb 1.
Antidiabetic potential of phycocyanin: effects on KKAy mice.

Indian J Med Res. 2012 Mar;135:422-8.
Alleviation of metabolic abnormalities induced by excessive fructose administration in Wistar rats by Spirulina maxima.
Jarouliya U1, Zacharia JA, Kumar P, Bisen PS, Prasad GB.

Association of glycaemia with macrovascular and microvascular complications of type 2 diabetes (UKPDS 35): prospective observational study
BMJ 2000; 321 doi: http://dx.doi.org/10.1136/bmj.321.7258.405 (Published 12 August 2000)
Cite this as: BMJ 2000;321:405

Med Sci Sports Exerc. 2010 Jan;42(1):142-51. doi: 10.1249/MSS.0b013e3181ac7a45.
Ergogenic and antioxidant effects of spirulina supplementation in humans.
Kalafati M1, Jamurtas AZ, Nikolaidis MG, Paschalis V, Theodorou AA, Sakellariou GK, Koutedakis Y, Kouretas D.

Eur J Appl Physiol. 2006 Sep;98(2):220-6. Epub 2006 Aug 30.
Preventive effects of Spirulina platensis on skeletal muscle damage under exercise-induced oxidative stress.
Lu HK1, Hsieh CC, Hsu JJ, Yang YK, Chou HN.
Semin Hematol. 2008 Oct;45(4):225-34. doi: 10.1053/j.seminhematol.2008.07.009.
Nutritional anemias and the elderly.
Carmel R1.

Cell Mol Immunol. 2011 May; 8(3): 248–254.
Published online 2011 Jan 31. doi: 10.1038/cmi.2010.76
PMCID: PMC4012879
The effects of Spirulina on anemia and immune function in senior citizens
Carlo Selmi,1,2 Patrick SC Leung,1 Laura Fischer,3 Bruce German,3 Chen-Yen Yang,1 Thomas P Kenny,1 Gerry R Cysewski,4 and M Eric Gershwin1
ISRN Allergy. 2013 Nov 13;2013:938751. doi: 10.1155/2013/938751. eCollection 2013.
Complementary therapies in allergic rhinitis.
Sayin I1, Cingi C, Oghan F, Baykal B, Ulusoy S.

J Sci Food Agric. 2014 Feb;94(3):432-7. doi: 10.1002/jsfa.6261.
Epub 2013 Jul 10.

The hypolipidaemic effects of Spirulina (Arthrospira platensis) supplementation in a Cretan population: a prospective study.
Mazokopakis EE1, Starakis IK, Papadomanolaki MG, Mavroeidi NG, Ganotakis ES.
Lipids Health Dis. 2007; 6: 33.
Published online 2007 Nov 26. doi: 10.1186/1476-511X-6-33
PMCID: PMC2211748

Antihyperlipemic and antihypertensive effects of Spirulina maxima in an open sample of mexican population: a preliminary report
Patricia V Torres-Duran,1 Aldo Ferreira-Hermosillo,1 and Marco A Juarez-Oropezacorresponding author1
Int J Biol Sci. 2009; 5(4): 377–387.
Published online 2009 Jun 2.
PMCID: PMC2695150

Chemoprevention of rat liver toxicity and carcinogenesis by Spirulina
Mohamed F Ismail,3 Doaa A Ali,3 Augusta Fernando,1 Mohamed E Abdraboh,1 Rajiv L Gaur,1 Wael M Ibrahim,3 Madhwa HG Raj,2 and Allal Ouhtit1,3,
Nutr Res Pract. 2008 Winter; 2(4): 295–300.
Published online 2008 Dec 31. doi: 10.4162/nrp.2008.2.4.295
PMCID: PMC2788188

A randomized study to establish the effects of spirulina in type 2 diabetes mellitus patients
Eun Hee Lee,1 Ji-Eun Park,1 Young-Ju Choi,2 Kap-Bum Huh,2 and Wha-Young Kimcorresponding author1
J Med Food. 2001 Winter;4(4):193-199.

Role of Spirulina in the Control of Glycemia and Lipidemia in Type 2 Diabetes Mellitus.
Parikh P1, Mani U, Iyer U.
J Sci Food Agric. 2014 Feb;94(3):432-7. doi: 10.1002/jsfa.6261.
Epub 2013 Jul 10.

The hypolipidaemic effects of Spirulina (Arthrospira platensis) supplementation in a Cretan population: a prospective study.
Mazokopakis EE1, Starakis IK, Papadomanolaki MG, Mavroeidi NG, Ganotakis ES.
J Appl Microbiol. 2009 Nov;107(5):1763; author reply 1764. doi: 10.1111/j.1365-2672.2009.04468.x. Epub 2009 Jul 13.

The evidence that pseudovitamin B(12) is biologically active in mammals is still lacking - a comment on Molina et al.'s (2009) experimental design.
Santos F, Teusink B, de Vos WM, Hugenholtz J.

Gut Health

Abrahamsson TR, Jakobsson T, Bottcher MF, Fredrikson M, Jenmalm MC, Bjorksten B, Oldaeus G. Probiotics in prevention of IgE-associated eczema: a double-blind, randomized, placebo-controlled trial. J Allergy Clin Immunol 119: 1174–1180, 2007.

Aggarwal BB, Kumar A, Bharti AC. Anticancer potential of curcumin: preclinical and clinical studies. Anticancer Res 23: 363–398, 2003.

Alakomi HL, Skytta E, Saarela M, Mattila-Sandholm T, Latva-Kala K, Helander IM. Lactic acid permeabilizes gram-negative bacteria by disrupting the outer membrane. Appl Environ Microbiol 66: 2001–2005, 2000.

Alam M, Midtvedt T, Uribe A. Differential cell kinetics in the ileum and colon of germfree rats. Scand J Gastroenterol 29: 445–451, 1994.

Alpert C, Scheel J, Engst W, Loh G, Blaut M. Adaptation of protein expression by Escherichia coli in the gastrointestinal tract of gnotobiotic mice. Environ Microbiol 11: 751–761, 2009.Medline

Amaral FA, Sachs D, Costa VV, Fagundes CT, Cisalpino D, Cunha TM, Ferreira SH, Cunha FQ, Silva TA, Nicoli JR, Vieira LQ, Souza DG, Teixeira MM. Commensal microbiota is fundamental for the development of inflammatory pain. Proc Natl Acad Sci USA 105: 2193–2197, 2008.

Antonopoulos DA, Huse SM, Morrison HG, Schmidt TM, Sogin ML, Young VB. Reproducible community dynamics of the gastrointestinal microbiota following antibiotic perturbation. Infect Immun 77: 2367–2375, 2009.

Atarashi K, Nishimura J, Shima T, Umesaki Y, Yamamoto M, Onoue M, Yagita H, Ishii N, Evans R, Honda K, Takeda K. ATP drives lamina propria T(H)17 cell differentiation. Nature 455: 808–812, 2008.

Backhed F, Ding H, Wang T, Hooper LV, Koh GY, Nagy A, Semenkovich CF, Gordon JI. The gut microbiota as an environmental factor that regulates fat storage. Proc Natl Acad Sci USA 101: 15718–15723, 2004.

Backhed F, Ley RE, Sonnenburg JL, Peterson DA, Gordon JI. Host-bacterial mutualism in the human intestine. Science 307: 1915–1920, 2005.

Balamurugan R, Janardhan HP, George S, Raghava MV, Muliyil J, Ramakrishna BS. Molecular studies of fecal anaerobic commensal bacteria in acute diarrhea in children. J Pediatr Gastroenterol Nutr 46: 514–519, 2008.

Banasaz M, Norin E, Holma R, Midtvedt T. Increased enterocyte production in gnotobiotic rats mono-associated with Lactobacillus rhamnosus GG. Appl Environ Microbiol 68: 3031–3034, 2002.

Barman M, Unold D, Shifley K, Amir E, Hung K, Bos N, Salzman N. Enteric salmonellosis disrupts the microbial ecology of the murine gastrointestinal tract. Infect Immun 76: 907–915, 2008.

Bartsch H, Nair J. Chronic inflammation and oxidative stress in the genesis and perpetuation of cancer: role of lipid peroxidation, DNA damage, and repair. Langenbecks Arch Surg 391: 499–510, 2006.

Bassi C, Larvin M, Villatoro E. Antibiotic therapy for prophylaxis against infection of pancreatic necrosis in acute pancreatitis. Cochrane Database Syst Rev CD002941, 2003.

Bates JM, Akerlund J, Mittge E, Guillemin K. Intestinal alkaline phosphatase detoxifies lipopolysaccharide and prevents inflammation in zebrafish in response to the gut microbiota. Cell Host Microbe 2: 371–382, 2007.

Beutler B, Rietschel ET. Innate immune sensing and its roots: the story of endotoxin. Nat Rev Immunol 3: 169–176, 2003.

Bik EM, Eckburg PB, Gill SR, Nelson KE, Purdom EA, Francois F, Perez-Perez G, Blaser MJ, Relman DA. Molecular analysis of the bacterial microbiota in the human stomach. Proc Natl Acad Sci USA 103: 732–737, 2006.

Bingham SA. Diet and colorectal cancer prevention. Biochem Soc Trans 28: 12–16, 2000.

Bjorksten B, Sepp E, Julge K, Voor T, Mikelsaar M. Allergy development and the intestinal microflora during the first year of life. J Allergy Clin Immunol 108: 516–520, 2001.

Bolte ER. Autism and Clostridium tetani. Med Hypotheses 51: 133–144, 1998.

Bouma G, Strober W. The immunological and genetic basis of inflammatory bowel disease. Nat Rev Immunol 3: 521–533, 2003.

Bourriaud C, Akoka S, Goupry S, Robins R, Cherbut C, Michel C. Butyrate production from lactate by human colonic microflora. Reprod Nutr Dev 42: S55, 2002.

Bouskra D, Brezillon C, Berard M, Werts C, Varona R, Boneca IG, Eberl G. Lymphoid tissue genesis induced by commensals through NOD1 regulates intestinal homeostasis. Nature 456: 507–510, 2008.

Brandl K, Plitas G, Mihu CN, Ubeda C, Jia T, Fleisher M, Schnabl B, DeMatteo RP, Pamer EG. Vancomycin-resistant enterococci exploit antibiotic-induced innate immune deficits. Nature 455: 804–807, 2008.

Brugman S, Klatter FA, Visser JT, Wildeboer-Veloo AC, Harmsen HJ, Rozing J, Bos NA. Antibiotic treatment partially protects against type 1 diabetes in the Bio-Breeding diabetes-prone rat. Is the gut flora involved in the development of type 1 diabetes? Diabetologia 49: 2105–2108, 2006.

Bry L, Falk PG, Midtvedt T, Gordon JI. A model of host-microbial interactions in an open mammalian ecosystem. Science 273: 1380–1383, 1996.

Bukowska H, Pieczul-Mroz J, Jastrzebska M, Chelstowski K, Naruszewicz M. Decrease in fibrinogen and LDL-cholesterol levels upon supplementation of diet with Lactobacillus plantarum in subjects with moderately elevated cholesterol. Atherosclerosis 137: 437–438, 1998.

Businco L, Bellanti J. Food allergy in childhood. Hypersensitivity to cows' milk allergens. Clin Exp Allergy 23: 481–483, 1993.

Calcinaro F, Dionisi S, Marinaro M, Candeloro P, Bonato V, Marzotti S, Corneli RB, Ferretti E, Gulino A, Grasso F, De Simone C, Di Mario U, Falorni A, Boirivant M, Dotta F. Oral probiotic administration induces interleukin-10 production and prevents spontaneous autoimmune diabetes in the non-obese diabetic mouse. Diabetologia 48: 1565–1575, 2005.

Caldarella MP, Giamberardino MA, Sacco F, Affaitati G, Milano A, Lerza R, Balatsinou C, Laterza F, Pierdomenico SD, Cuccurullo F, Neri M. Sensitivity disturbances in patients with irritable bowel syndrome and fibromyalgia. Am J Gastroenterol 101: 2782–2789, 2006.

Cario E, Gerken G, Podolsky DK. Toll-like receptor 2 controls mucosal inflammation by regulating epithelial barrier function. Gastroenterology 132: 1359–1374, 2007.

Cash HL, Whitham CV, Behrendt CL, Hooper LV. Symbiotic bacteria direct expression of an intestinal bactericidal lectin. Science 313: 1126–1130, 2006.

Celli J, Deng W, Finlay BB. Enteropathogenic Escherichia coli (EPEC) attachment to epithelial cells: exploiting the host cell cytoskeleton from the outside. Cell Microbiol 2: 1–9, 2000.CrossRefMedlineWeb of Science

Chang JY, Antonopoulos DA, Kalra A, Tonelli A, Khalife WT, Schmidt TM, Young VB. Decreased diversity of the fecal Microbiome in recurrent Clostridium difficile-associated diarrhea. J Infect Dis 197: 435–438, 2008.

Chen YC, Eisner JD, Kattar MM, Rassoulian-Barrett SL, Lafe K, Bui U, Limaye AP, Cookson BT. Polymorphic internal transcribed spacer region 1 DNA sequences identify medically important yeasts. J Clin Microbiol 39: 4042–4051, 2001.

Chiller K, Selkin BA, Murakawa GJ. Skin microflora and bacterial infections of the skin. J Invest Dermatol Symp Proc 6: 170–174, 2001.

Christensen HR, Frokiaer H, Pestka JJ. Lactobacilli differentially modulate expression of cytokines and maturation surface markers in murine dendritic cells. J Immunol 168: 171–178, 2002.

Churruca I, Fernandez-Quintela A, Portillo MP. Conjugated linoleic acid isomers: differences in metabolism and biological effects. Biofactors 35: 105–111, 2009.

Clarke MB, Hughes DT, Zhu C, Boedeker EC, Sperandio V. The QseC sensor kinase: a bacterial adrenergic receptor. Proc Natl Acad Sci USA 103: 10420–10425, 2006.

Collins SM, Bercik P. The relationship between intestinal microbiota and the central nervous system in normal gastrointestinal function and disease. Gastroenterology 136: 2003–2014, 2009.

Corr SC, Gahan CG, Hill C. Impact of selected Lactobacillus and Bifidobacterium species on Listeria monocytogenes infection and the mucosal immune response. FEMS Immunol Med Microbiol 50: 380–388, 2007.

Correa P, Houghton J. Carcinogenesis of Helicobacter pylori. Gastroenterology 133: 659–672, 2007.

Crawford PA, Crowley JR, Sambandam N, Muegge BD, Costello EK, Hamady M, Knight R, Gordon JI. Regulation of myocardial ketone body metabolism by the gut microbiota during nutrient deprivation. Proc Natl Acad Sci USA 106: 11276–11281, 2009.

Croswell A, Amir E, Teggatz P, Barman M, Salzman NH. Prolonged impact of antibiotics on intestinal microbial ecology and susceptibility to enteric Salmonella infection. Infect Immun 77: 2741–2753, 2009.

Dabard J, Bridonneau C, Phillipe C, Anglade P, Molle D, Nardi M, Ladire M, Girardin H, Marcille F, Gomez A, Fons M. Ruminococcin A, a new antibiotic produced by a Ruminococcus gnavus strain isolated from human feces. Appl Environ Microbiol 67: 4111–4118, 2001.

De La Cochetiere MF, Durand T, Lalande V, Petit JC, Potel G, Beaugerie L. Effect of antibiotic therapy on human fecal microbiota and the relation to the development of Clostridium difficile. Microb Ecol 56: 395–402, 2008.

De Madaria E, Martinez J, Lozano B, Sempere L, Benlloch S, Such J, Uceda F, Frances R, Perez-Mateo M. Detection and identification of bacterial DNA in serum from patients with acute pancreatitis. Gut 54: 1293–1297, 2005.

57.↵ Destoumieux-Garzon D, Peduzzi J, Rebuffat S. Focus on modified microcins: structural features and mechanisms of action. Biochimie 84: 511–519, 2002.CrossRefMedlineWeb of Science

Dethlefsen L, Huse S, Sogin ML, Relman DA. The pervasive effects of an antibiotic on the human gut microbiota, as revealed by deep 16S rRNA sequencing. PLoS Biol 6: e280, 2008.

Dubos RJ, Savage DC, Schaedler RW. The indigenous flora of the gastrointestinal tract. Dis Colon Rectum 10: 23–34, 1967.

Duncan SH, Louis P, Flint HJ. Cultivable bacterial diversity from the human colon. Lett Appl Microbiol 44: 343–350, 2007.

Duncan SH, Louis P, Flint HJ. Lactate-utilizing bacteria, isolated from human feces, that produce butyrate as a major fermentation product. Appl Environ Microbiol 70: 5810–5817, 2004.

Eckburg PB, Bik EM, Bernstein CN, Purdom E, Dethlefsen L, Sargent M, Gill SR, Nelson KE, Relman DA. Diversity of the human intestinal microbial flora. Science 308: 1635–1638, 2005.

Eisenhofer G, Aneman A, Friberg P, Hooper D, Fandriks L, Lonroth H, Hunyady B, Mezey E. Substantial production of dopamine in the human gastrointestinal tract. J Clin Endocrinol Metab 82: 3864–3871, 1997.

Falk PG, Hooper LV, Midtvedt T, Gordon JI. Creating and maintaining the gastrointestinal ecosystem: what we know and need to know from gnotobiology. Microbiol Mol Biol Rev 62: 1157–1170, 1998.

Feleszko W, Jaworska J, Rha RD, Steinhausen S, Avagyan A, Jaudszus A, Ahrens B, Groneberg DA, Wahn U, Hamelmann E. Probiotic-induced suppression of allergic sensitization and airway inflammation is associated with an increase of T regulatory-dependent mechanisms in a murine model of asthma. Clin Exp Allergy 37: 498–505, 2007.

Fetissov SO, Hamze Sinno M, Coeffier M, Bole-Feysot C, Ducrotte P, Hokfelt T, Dechelotte P. Autoantibodies against appetite-regulating peptide hormones and neuropeptides: putative modulation by gut microflora. Nutrition 24: 348–359, 2008.

Fetissov SO, Hamze Sinno M, Coquerel Q, Do Rego JC, Coeffier M, Gilbert D, Hokfelt T, Dechelotte P. Emerging role of autoantibodies against appetite-regulating neuropeptides in eating disorders. Nutrition 24: 854–859, 2008.

Finegold SM. Therapy and epidemiology of autism–clostridial spores as key elements. Med Hypotheses 70: 508–511, 2008.

Finegold SM, Molitoris D, Song Y, Liu C, Vaisanen ML, Bolte E, McTeague M, Sandler R, Wexler H, Marlowe EM, Collins MD, Lawson PA, Summanen P, Baysallar M, Tomzynski TJ, Read E, Johnson E, Rolfe R, Nasir P, Shah H, Haake DA, Manning P, Kaul A. Gastrointestinal microflora studies in late-onset autism. Clin Infect Dis 35: S6–S16, 2002.

Fink LN, Zeuthen LH, Christensen HR, Morandi B, Frokiaer H, Ferlazzo G. Distinct gut-derived lactic acid bacteria elicit divergent dendritic cell-mediated NK cell responses. Int Immunol 19: 1319–1327, 2007.

Forsythe P, Inman MD, Bienenstock J. Oral treatment with live Lactobacillus reuteri inhibits the allergic airway response in mice. Am J Respir Crit Care Med 175: 561–569, 2007.

Gebbers JO, Laissue JA. Immunologic structures and functions of the gut. Schweiz Arch Tierheilkd 131: 221–238, 1989.

Giannakis M, Chen SL, Karam SM, Engstrand L, Gordon JI. Helicobacter pylori evolution during progression from chronic atrophic gastritis to gastric cancer and its impact on gastric stem cells. Proc Natl Acad Sci USA 105: 4358–4363, 2008.

Hooper LV, Gordon JI. Commensal host-bacterial relationships in the gut. Science 292: 1115–1118, 2001.

Hooper LV, Stappenbeck TS, Hong CV, Gordon JI. Angiogenins: a new class of microbicidal proteins involved in innate immunity. Nat Immunol 4: 269–273, 2003.

Hooper LV, Wong MH, Thelin A, Hansson L, Falk PG, Gordon JI. Molecular analysis of commensal host-microbial relationships in the intestine. Science 291: 881–884, 2001.

Huurre A, Kalliomaki M, Rautava S, Rinne M, Salminen S, Isolauri E. Mode of delivery: effects on gut microbiota and humoral immunity. Neonatology 93: 236–240, 2008.CrossRefMedlineWeb of Science

Huycke MM, Abrams V, Moore DR. Enterococcus faecalis produces extracellular superoxide and hydrogen peroxide that damages colonic epithelial cell DNA. Carcinogenesis 23: 529–536, 2002.

Hviid A, Svanstrom H. Antibiotic use and intussusception in early childhood. J Antimicrob Chemother 64: 642–648, 2009.

Iapichino G, Callegari ML, Marzorati S, Cigada M, Corbella D, Ferrari S, Morelli L. Impact of antibiotics on the gut microbiota of critically ill patients. J Med Microbiol 57: 1007–1014, 2008.

Jernberg C, Lofmark S, Edlund C, Jansson JK. Long-term ecological impacts of antibiotic administration on the human intestinal microbiota. Isme J 1: 56–66, 2007.

Kalliomaki M, Kirjavainen P, Eerola E, Kero P, Salminen S, Isolauri E. Distinct patterns of neonatal gut microflora in infants in whom atopy was and was not developing. J Allergy Clin Immunol 107: 129–134, 2001.

Kalliomaki M, Salminen S, Arvilommi H, Kero P, Koskinen P, Isolauri E. Probiotics in primary prevention of atopic disease: a randomised placebo-controlled trial. Lancet 357: 1076–1079, 2001.

Kanehisa M, Goto S, Kawashima S, Okuno Y, Hattori M. The KEGG resource for deciphering the genome. Nucleic Acids Res 32: D277–D280, 2004.

Karra E, Batterham RL. The role of gut hormones in the regulation of body weight and energy homeostasis. Mol Cell Endocrinol 316: 120–128, 2009.

Kopp MV, Hennemuth I, Heinzmann A, Urbanek R. Randomized, double-blind, placebo-controlled trial of probiotics for primary prevention: no clinical effects of Lactobacillus GG supplementation. Pediatrics 121: e850–e856, 2008.

Kurokawa K, Itoh T, Kuwahara T, Oshima K, Toh H, Toyoda A, Takami H, Morita H, Sharma VK, Srivastava TP, Taylor TD, Noguchi H, Mori H, Ogura Y, Ehrlich DS, Itoh K, Takagi T, Sakaki Y, Hayashi T, Hattori M. Comparative metagenomics revealed commonly enriched gene sets in human gut microbiomes. DNA Res 14: 169–181, 2007.

Ley RE, Backhed F, Turnbaugh P, Lozupone CA, Knight RD, Gordon JI. Obesity alters gut microbial ecology. Proc Natl Acad Sci USA 102: 11070–11075, 2005.

Ley RE, Peterson DA, Gordon JI. Ecological and evolutionary forces shaping microbial diversity in the human intestine. Cell 124: 837–848, 2006.

Ramzy PI, Wolf SE, Irtun O, Hart DW, Thompson JC, Herndon DN. Gut epithelial apoptosis after severe burn: effects of gut hypoperfusion. J Am Coll Surg 190: 281–287, 2000.

Rhee SH, Pothoulakis C, Mayer EA. Principles and clinical implications of the brain-gut-enteric microbiota axis. Nat Rev Gastroenterol Hepatol 6: 306–314, 2009.

Roth KA, Kapadia SB, Martin SM, Lorenz RG. Cellular immune responses are essential for the development of Helicobacter felis-associated gastric pathology. J Immunol 163: 1490–1497, 1999.

Russell WR, Scobbie L, Chesson A, Richardson AJ, Stewart CS, Duncan SH, Drew JE, Duthie GG. Anti-inflammatory implications of the microbial transformation of dietary phenolic compounds. Nutr Cancer 60: 636–642, 2008.

Ryan CM, Yarmush ML, Burke JF, Tompkins RG. Increased gut permeability early after burns correlates with the extent of burn injury. Crit Care Med 20: 1508–1512, 1992.

Salminen S, Isolauri E. Intestinal colonization, microbiota and probiotics. J Pediatr 149: S115–S120, 2006.

Sandler RH, Finegold SM, Bolte ER, Buchanan CP, Maxwell AP, Vaisanen ML, Nelson MN, Wexler HM. Short-term benefit from oral vancomycin treatment of regressive-onset autism. J Child Neurol 15: 429–435, 2000.

Sanz Y, Nadal I, Sanchez E. Probiotics as drugs against human gastrointestinal infections. Recent Patents Anti-Infect Drug Disc 2: 148–156, 2007.

Sartor RB. Mechanisms of disease: pathogenesis of Crohn's disease and ulcerative colitis. Nat Clin Pract Gastroenterol Hepatol 3: 390–407, 2006.

Sartor RB. Microbial influences in inflammatory bowel diseases. Gastroenterology 134: 577–594, 2008.

Savage DC. Associations of indigenous microorganisms with gastrointestinal mucosal epithelia. Am J Clin Nutr 23: 1495–1501, 1970.

Savage DC. Microbial ecology of the gastrointestinal tract. Annu Rev Microbiol 31: 107–133, 1977.

Scanlan PD, Shanahan F, Clune Y, Collins JK, O'Sullivan GC, O'Riordan M, Holmes E, Wang Y, Marchesi JR. Culture-independent analysis of the gut microbiota in colorectal cancer and polyposis. Environ Microbiol 10: 789–798, 2008.

Schwartz RF, Neu J, Schatz D, Atkinson MA, Wasserfall C. Comment on: Brugman S et al. (2006) Antibiotic treatment partially protects against type 1 diabetes in the Bio-Breeding diabetes-prone rat. Is the gut flora involved in the development of type 1 diabetes? Diabetologia 49: 2105–2108. Diabetologia 50: 220–221, 2007.

Sekirov I, Finlay BB. The role of the intestinal microbiota in enteric infection. J Physiol 587: 4159–4167, 2009.

Sekirov I, Tam NM, Jogova M, Robertson ML, Li Y, Lupp C, Finlay BB. Antibiotic-induced perturbations of the intestinal microbiota alter host susceptibility to enteric infection. Infect Immun 76: 4726–4736, 2008.

Shimizu K, Ogura H, Goto M, Asahara T, Nomoto K, Morotomi M, Yoshiya K, Matsushima A, Sumi Y, Kuwagata Y, Tanaka H, Shimazu T, Sugimoto H. Altered gut flora and environment in patients with severe SIRS. J Trauma 60: 126–133, 2006.

Sidhu H, Allison MJ, Chow JM, Clark A, Peck AB. Rapid reversal of hyperoxaluria in a rat model after probiotic administration of Oxalobacter formigenes. J Urol 166: 1487–1491, 2001.

Sjogren YM, Jenmalm MC, Bottcher MF, Bjorksten B, Sverremark-Ekstrom E. Altered early infant gut microbiota in children developing allergy up to 5 years of age. Clin Exp Allergy 39: 518–526, 2009.

Smith NR, Kishchuk BE, Mohn WW. Effects of wildfire and harvest disturbances on forest soil bacterial communities. Appl Environ Microbiol 74: 216–224, 2008.

Sokol H, Pigneur B, Watterlot L, Lakhdari O, Bermudez-Humaran LG, Gratadoux JJ, Blugeon S, Bridonneau C, Furet JP, Corthier G, Grangette C, Vasquez N, Pochart P, Trugnan G, Thomas G, Blottiere HM, Dore J, Marteau P, Seksik P, Langella P. Faecalibacterium prausnitzii is an anti-inflammatory commensal bacterium identified by gut microbiota analysis of Crohn disease patients. Proc Natl Acad Sci USA 105: 16731–16736, 2008.

Song Y, Liu C, Finegold SM. Real-time PCR quantitation of clostridia in feces of autistic children. Appl Environ Microbiol 70: 6459–6465, 2004.

Sonnenburg JL, Xu J, Leip DD, Chen CH, Westover BP, Weatherford J, Buhler JD, Gordon JI. Glycan foraging in vivo by an intestine-adapted bacterial symbiont. Science 307: 1955–1959, 2005.

Sperandio V, Mellies JL, Nguyen W, Shin S, Kaper JB. Quorum sensing controls expression of the type III secretion gene transcription and protein secretion in enterohemorrhagic and enteropathogenic Escherichia coli. Proc Natl Acad Sci USA 96: 15196–15201, 1999.

Sperandio V, Torres AG, Giron JA, Kaper JB. Quorum sensing is a global regulatory mechanism in enterohemorrhagic Escherichia coli O157:H7. J Bacteriol 183: 5187–5197, 2001.

Sperandio V, Torres AG, Jarvis B, Nataro JP, Kaper JB. Bacteria-host communication: the language of hormones. Proc Natl Acad Sci USA 100: 8951–8956, 2003.

Sperandio V, Torres AG, Kaper JB. Quorum sensing Escherichia coli regulators B and C (QseBC): a novel two-component regulatory system involved in the regulation of flagella and motility by quorum sensing in E. coli. Mol Microbiol 43: 809–821, 2002.

Spiller R, Garsed K. Postinfectious irritable bowel syndrome. Gastroenterology 136: 1979–1988, 2009.

Srikanth CV, McCormick BA. Interactions of the intestinal epithelium with the pathogen and the indigenous microbiota: a three-way crosstalk. Interdiscip Perspect Infect Dis 2008: 626–827, 2008.

Stappenbeck TS, Hooper LV, Gordon JI. Developmental regulation of intestinal angiogenesis by indigenous microbes via Paneth cells. Proc Natl Acad Sci USA 99: 15451–15455, 2002.

Stecher B, Barthel M, Schlumberger MC, Haberli L, Rabsch W, Kremer M, Hardt WD. Motility allows S. typhimurium to benefit from the mucosal defence. Cell Microbiol 10: 1166–1180, 2008.

Stecher B, Hardt WD. The role of microbiota in infectious disease. Trends Microbiol 16: 107–114, 2008.

Stecher B, Robbiani R, Walker AW, Westendorf AM, Barthel M, Kremer M, Chaffron S, Macpherson AJ, Buer J, Parkhill J, Dougan G, von Mering C, Hardt WD. Salmonella enterica serovar typhimurium exploits inflammation to compete with the intestinal microbiota. PLoS Biol 5: 2177–2189, 2007.

Stehr M, Greweling MC, Tischer S, Singh M, Blocker H, Monner DA, Muller W. Charles River altered Schaedler flora [CRASF(R)] remained stable for four years in a mouse colony housed in individually ventilated cages. Lab Anim 43: 362–370, 2009.

Strachan DP. Family size, infection and atopy: the first decade of the "hygiene hypothesis." Thorax 55 Suppl 1: S2–S10, 2000.

Strachan DP. Hay fever, hygiene, and household size. BMJ 299: 1259–1260, 1989.

Sudo N. Stress and gut microbiota: does postnatal microbial colonization programs the hypothalamic-pituitary-adrenal system for stress response? Int Congr Ser 1287: 350–354, 2006.

Sudo N, Chida Y, Aiba Y, Sonoda J, Oyama N, Yu XN, Kubo C, Koga Y. Postnatal microbial colonization programs the hypothalamic-pituitary-adrenal system for stress response in mice. J Physiol 558: 263–275, 2004.CrossRefMedline

Sundquist A, Bigdeli S, Jalili R, Druzin ML, Waller S, Pullen KM, El-Sayed YY, Taslimi MM, Batzoglou S, Ronaghi M. Bacterial flora-typing with targeted, chip-based Pyrosequencing. BMC Microbiol 7: 108,

Surawicz CM, McFarland LV, Greenberg RN, Rubin M, Fekety R, Mulligan ME, Garcia RJ, Brandmarker S, Bowen K, Borjal D, Elmer GW. The search for a better treatment for recurrent Clostridium difficile disease: use of high-dose vancomycin combined with Saccharomyces boulardii. Clin Infect Dis 31: 1012–1017, 2000.

Suzuki K, Meek B, Doi Y, Muramatsu M, Chiba T, Honjo T, Fagarasan S. Aberrant expansion of segmented filamentous bacteria in IgA-deficient gut. Proc Natl Acad Sci USA 101: 1981–1986, 2004.

Suzuki S, Shimojo N, Tajiri Y, Kumemura M, Kohno Y. A quantitative and relative increase in intestinal bacteroides in allergic infants in rural Japan. Asian Pac J Allergy Immunol 26: 113–119, 2008.

Swann J, Wang Y, Abecia L, Costabile A, Tuohy K, Gibson G, Roberts D, Sidaway J, Jones H, Wilson ID, Nicholson J, Holmes E. Gut microbiome modulates the toxicity of hydrazine: a metabonomic study. Mol Biosyst 5: 351–355, 2009.

Swidsinski A, Loening-Baucke V, Lochs H, Hale LP. Spatial organization of bacterial flora in normal and inflamed intestine: a fluorescence in situ hybridization study in mice. World J Gastroenterol 11: 1131–1140, 2005.

Tanaka S, Kobayashi T, Songjinda P, Tateyama A, Tsubouchi M, Kiyohara C, Shirakawa T, Sonomoto K, Nakayama J. Influence of antibiotic exposure in the early postnatal period on the development of intestinal microbiota. FEMS Immunol Med Microbiol 56: 80–87, 2009.

Taylor AL, Dunstan JA, Prescott SL. Probiotic supplementation for the first 6 months of life fails to reduce the risk of atopic dermatitis and increases the risk of allergen sensitization in high-risk children: a randomized controlled trial. J Allergy Clin Immunol 119: 184–191, 2007.CrossRefMedlineWeb of Science

Termen S, Tollin M, Rodriguez E, Sveinsdottir SH, Johannesson B, Cederlund A, Sjovall J, Agerberth B, Gudmundsson GH. PU1 and bacterial metabolites regulate the human gene CAMP encoding antimicrobial peptide LL-37 in colon epithelial cells. Mol Immunol 45: 3947–3955, 2008.

Tsuji M, Suzuki K, Kinoshita K, Fagarasan S. Dynamic interactions between bacteria and immune cells leading to intestinal IgA synthesis. Semin Immunol 20: 59–66, 2008.

Turnbaugh PJ, Backhed F, Fulton L, Gordon JI. Diet-induced obesity is linked to marked but reversible alterations in the mouse distal gut microbiome. Cell Host Microbe 3: 213–223, 2008.

Turnbaugh PJ, Hamady M, Yatsunenko T, Cantarel BL, Duncan A, Ley RE, Sogin ML, Jones WJ, Roe BA, Affourtit JP, Egholm M, Henrissat B, Heath AC, Knight R, Gordon JI. A core gut microbiome in obese and lean twins. Nature 457: 480–484, 2009.

Turnbaugh PJ, Ley RE, Mahowald MA, Magrini V, Mardis ER, Gordon JI. An obesity-associated gut microbiome with increased capacity for energy harvest. Nature 444: 1027–1031, 2006.

Uronis JM, Muhlbauer M, Herfarth HH, Rubinas TC, Jones GS, Jobin C. Modulation of the intestinal microbiota alters colitis-associated colorectal cancer susceptibility. PLoS One 4: e6026, 2009.

Vaishnava S, Behrendt CL, Ismail AS, Eckmann L, Hooper LV. Paneth cells directly sense gut commensals and maintain homeostasis at the intestinal host-microbial interface. Proc Natl Acad Sci USA 105: 20858–20863, 2008.

Vella A, Farrugia G. d-Lactic acidosis: pathologic consequence of saprophytism. Mayo Clin Proc 73: 451–456, 1998.

Verberkmoes NC, Russell AL, Shah M, Godzik A, Rosenquist M, Halfvarson J, Lefsrud MG, Apajalahti J, Tysk C, Hettich RL, Jansson JK. Shotgun metaproteomics of the human distal gut microbiota. ISME J 3: 179–189, 2009.

Verhulst SL, Vael C, Beunckens C, Nelen V, Goossens H, Desager K. A longitudinal analysis on the association between antibiotic use, intestinal microflora, and wheezing during the first year of life. J Asthma 45: 828–832, 2008.

Verstraelen H. Cutting edge: the vaginal microflora and bacterial vaginosis. Verh K Acad Geneeskd Belg 70: 147–174, 2008

Von Mering C, Jensen LJ, Kuhn M, Chaffron S, Doerks T, Kruger B, Snel B, Bork P. STRING 7–recent developments in the integration and prediction of protein interactions. Nucleic Acids Res 35: D358–D362, 2007.

Wagner CL, Taylor SN, Johnson D. Host factors in amniotic fluid and breast milk that contribute to gut maturation. Clin Rev Allergy Immunol 34: 191–204, 2008.

Wang Z, Xiao G, Yao Y, Guo S, Lu K, Sheng Z. The role of bifidobacteria in gut barrier function after thermal injury in rats. J Trauma 61: 650–657,

Wen L, Ley RE, Volchkov PY, Stranges PB, Avanesyan L, Stonebraker AC, Hu C, Wong FS, Szot GL, Bluestone JA, Gordon JI, Chervonsky AV. Innate immunity and intestinal microbiota in the development of Type 1 diabetes. Nature 455: 1109–1113, 2008.

Weston S, Halbert A, Richmond P, Prescott SL. Effects of probiotics on atopic dermatitis: a randomised controlled trial. Arch Dis Child 90: 892–897, 2005.

Whary MT, Danon SJ, Feng Y, Ge Z, Sundina N, Ng V, Taylor NS, Rogers AB, Fox JG. Rapid onset of ulcerative typhlocolitis in B6.129P2-IL10tm1Cgn (IL-10-/-) mice infected with Helicobacter trogontum is associated with decreased colonization by altered Schaedler's flora. Infect Immun 74: 6615–6623, 2006.

White JS, Hoper M, Parks RW, Clements WD, Diamond T. Patterns of bacterial translocation in experimental biliary obstruction. J Surg Res 132: 80–84,

Whitehead WE, Palsson O, Jones KR. Systematic review of the comorbidity of irritable bowel syndrome with other disorders: what are the causes and implications? Gastroenterology 122: 1140–1156, 2002.

Whitman WB, Coleman DC, Wiebe WJ. Prokaryotes: the unseen majority. Proc Natl Acad Sci USA 95: 6578–6583, 1998.

Wikoff WR, Anfora AT, Liu J, Schultz PG, Lesley SA, Peters EC, Siuzdak G. Metabolomics analysis reveals large effects of gut microflora on mammalian blood metabolites. Proc Natl Acad Sci USA 106: 3698–3703, 2009.

Willing B, Halfvarson J, Dicksved J, Rosenquist M, Jarnerot G, Engstrand L, Tysk C, Jansson JK. Twin studies reveal specific imbalances in the mucosa-associated microbiota of patients with ileal Crohn's disease. Inflamm Bowel Dis 15: 653–660, 2009.

Wjst M, Hoelscher B, Frye C, Wichmann HE, Dold S, Heinrich J. Early antibiotic treatment and later asthma. Eur J Med Res 6: 263–271, 2001.MedlineWeb of Science

Wostmann BS, Wiech NL, Kung E. Catabolism and elimination of cholesterol in germfree rats. J Lipid Res 7: 77–82, 1966.

Xavier RJ, Podolsky DK. Unravelling the pathogenesis of inflammatory bowel disease. Nature 448: 427–434, 2007.CrossRefMedlineWeb of Science

Xu J, Gordon JI. Inaugural article: honor thy symbionts. Proc Natl Acad Sci USA 100: 10452–10459, 2003.

Xu J, Mahowald MA, Ley RE, Lozupone CA, Hamady M, Martens EC, Henrissat B, Coutinho PM, Minx P, Latreille P, Cordum H, Van Brunt A, Kim K, Fulton RS, Fulton LA, Clifton SW, Wilson RK, Knight RD, Gordon JI. Evolution of symbiotic bacteria in the distal human intestine. PLoS Biol 5: e156, 2007.

Yanagibashi T, Hosono A, Oyama A, Tsuda M, Hachimura S, Takahashi Y, Itoh K, Hirayama K, Takahashi K, Kaminogawa S. Bacteroides induce higher IgA production than lactobacillus by increasing activation-induced cytidine deaminase expression in B cells in murine Peyer's patches. Biosci Biotechnol Biochem 73: 372–377, 2009.

Yap IK, Li JV, Saric J, Martin FP, Davies H, Wang Y, Wilson ID, Nicholson JK, Utzinger J, Marchesi JR, Holmes E. Metabonomic and microbiological analysis of the dynamic effect of vancomycin-induced gut microbiota modification in the mouse. J Proteome Res 7: 3718–3728, 2008.

Zaborina O, Lepine F, Xiao G, Valuckaite V, Chen Y, Li T, Ciancio M, Zaborin A, Petrof EO, Turner JR, Rahme LG, Chang E, Alverdy JC. Dynorphin activates quorum sensing quinolone signaling in Pseudomonas aeruginosa. PLoS Pathog 3: e35, 2007.

Zeuthen LH, Fink LN, Frokiaer H. Epithelial cells prime the immune response to an array of gut-derived commensals towards a tolerogenic phenotype through distinct actions of thymic stromal lymphopoietin and transforming growth factor-beta. Immunology 123: 197–208, 2008.

Zhang C, Zhang M, Wang S, Han R, Cao Y, Hua W, Mao Y, Zhang X, Pang X, Wei C, Zhao G, Chen Y, Zhao L. Interactions between gut microbiota, host genetics and diet relevant to development of metabolic syndromes in mice. ISME J 4: 232–241.

Zhang M, Zhang C, Du H, Wei G, Pang X, Zhou H, Liu B, Zhao L. Pattern extraction of structural responses of gut microbiota to rotavirus infection via multivariate statistical analysis of clone library data. FEMS Microbiol Ecol 70: 21–29, 2009.

Zhao HY, Wang HJ, Lu Z, Xu SZ. Intestinal microflora in patients with liver cirrhosis. Chin J Dig Dis 5: 64–67, 2004.

Zoetendal EG, Akkermans ADL, Akkermans-van Vliet WM, de Visser JAGM, de Vos WM. The host genotype affects the bacterial community in the human gastrointestinal tract. Micro Ecol Health Dis 13: 129–134, 2001.

Zoetendal EG, von Wright A, Vilpponen-Salmela T, Ben-Amor K, Akkermans AD, de Vos WM. Mucosa-associated bacteria in the human gastrointestinal tract are uniformly distributed along the colon and differ from the community recovered from feces. Appl Environ Microbiol 68: 3401–3407, 2002.

Seckl JR, Meaney MJ (2004) Glucocorticoid programming. Ann N Y Acad Sci 1032:63–84.

Ley RE, et al. (2008) Evolution of mammals and their gut microbes. Science 320:1647–1651.

Hooper LV, Gordon JI (2001) Commensal host-bacterial relationships in the gut. Science 292:1115–1118.

Lundin A, et al. (2008) Gut flora, Toll-like receptors and nuclear receptors: A tripartite communication that tunes innate immunity in large intestine. Cell Microbiol 10:1093–1103.

Björkholm B, et al. (2009) Intestinal microbiota regulate xenobiotic metabolism in the liver. PLoS ONE 4:e6958.

Claus SP, et al. (2008) Systemic multicompartmental effects of the gut microbiome on mouse metabolic phenotypes. Mol Syst Biol 4:219.

Gill SR, et al. (2006) Metagenomic analysis of the human distal gut microbiome. Science 312:1355–1359.

Finegold SM, et al. (2002) Gastrointestinal microflora studies in late-onset autism. Clin Infect Dis 35(Suppl 1):S6–S16.

↵ Mittal VA, Ellman LM, Cannon TD (2008) Gene-environment interaction and covariation in schizophrenia: The role of obstetric complications. Schizophr Bull 34:1083–1094.

Goehler LE, Park SM, Opitz N, Lyte M, Gaykema RP (2008) Campylobacter jejuni infection increases anxiety-like behavior in the holeboard: Possible anatomical substrates for viscerosensory modulation of exploratory behavior. Brain Behav Immun 22:354–366.

Bilbo SD, et al. (2005) Neonatal infection induces memory impairments following an immune challenge in adulthood. Behav Neurosci 119:293–301.

Sullivan R, et al. (2006) The International Society for Developmental Psychobiology annual meeting symposium: Impact of early life experiences on brain and behavioral development. Dev Psychobiol 48:583–602.

Desbonnet L, Garrett L, Clarke G, Bienenstock J, Dinan TG (2008) The probiotic Bifidobacteria infantis: An assessment of potential antidepressant properties in the rat. J Psychiatr Res 43:164–174.

Martinowich K, Manji H, Lu B (2007) New insights into BDNF function in depression and anxiety. Nat Neurosci 10:1089–1093.

Bateup HS, et al. (2010) Distinct subclasses of medium spiny neurons differentially regulate striatal motor behaviors. Proc Natl Acad Sci USA 107:14845–14850.

Sudo N, et al. (2004) Postnatal microbial colonization programs the hypothalamic-pituitary-adrenal system for stress response in mice. J Physiol 558:263–275.

Bäckhed F, Manchester JK, Semenkovich CF, Gordon JI (2007) Mechanisms underlying the resistance to diet-induced obesity in germ-free mice. Proc Natl Acad Sci USA 104:979–984.

Becher A, et al. (1999) The synaptophysin-synaptobrevin complex: A hallmark of synaptic vesicle maturation. J Neurosci 19:1922–1931.

Ulfig N, Setzer M, Neudörfer F, Bohl J (2000) Distribution of SNAP-25 in transient neuronal circuitries of the developing human forebrain. Neuroreport 11:1259–1263.

Borovikova LV, et al. (2000) Vagus nerve stimulation attenuates the systemic inflammatory response to endotoxin. Nature 405:458–462.

Wang X, et al. (2002) Evidences for vagus nerve in maintenance of immune balance and transmission of immune information from gut to brain in STM-infected rats. World J Gastroenterol 8:540–545.

Wikoff WR, et al. (2009) Metabolomics analysis reveals large effects of gut microflora on mammalian blood metabolites. Proc Natl Acad Sci USA 106:3698–3703.

Uribe A, Alam M, Johansson O, Midtvedt T, Theodorsson E (1994) Microflora modulates endocrine cells in the gastrointestinal mucosa of the rat. Gastroenterology 107:1259–1269.

Kawai M, Rosen CJ (2010) Minireview: A skeleton in serotonin's closet? Endocrinology 151:4103–4108.

Cools R, Roberts AC, Robbins TW (2008) Serotoninergic regulation of emotional and behavioural control processes. Trends Cogn Sci 12:31–40.

Aballay A (2009) Neural regulation of immunity: Role of NPR-1 in pathogen avoidance and regulation of innate immunity. Cell Cycle 8:966–969.

Laurin N, et al. (2008) Investigation of the G protein subunit Galphaolf gene (GNAL) in attention deficit/hyperactivity disorder. J Psychiatr Res 42:117–124.

Addolorato G, et al. (2008) State and trait anxiety and depression in patients affected by gastrointestinal diseases: Psychometric evaluation of 1641 patients referred to an internal medicine outpatient setting. Int J Clin Pract 62:1063–1069.

Nikolov RN, et al. (2009) Gastrointestinal symptoms in a sample of children with pervasive developmental disorders. J Autism Dev Disord 39:405–413.

Preventive Medicine
Volume 7, Issue 2, June 1978, Pages 205-217
Impact of westernization on the nutrition of Japanese: Changes in physique, cancer, longevity and centenarians Yasuo Kagawa

Walnuts

WebMD Health News, April 21, 2009
University of Maryland Medical Center, Alpha-linolenic acid
Nutr Metab Cardiovasc Dis. 2007 Jul;17(6):457-61.
J Med Food. 2011 Sep;14(9):890-8.
BMC Med. 2013 Jul 16;11:164.

World's Healthiest Foods, Walnuts
Phytochemistry Volume 63, Issue 7, August 2003, Pages 795–801
J Agric Food Chem. 2008 Jun 25;56(12):4444-9.
Food Funct. 2012 Feb;3(2):134-40.

American Journal of Clinical Nutrition April 17, 2013
Obesity (Silver Spring). 2010 Jun;18(6):1176-82.

Biology of Reproduction August 15, 2012
Br J Nutr. 2012 May;107(9):1393-401.
J Nutr. 2009 Sep;139(9):1813S-7S.

Eur J Clin Nutr. 2009 Aug;63(8):1008-15.
World's Healthiest Foods, Walnuts
nuthealth.org

Resources

Nutrition for Special Needs by Sue Cook
http://www.amazon.co.uk/Nutrition-Special-Needs-shall-brainbuzzz/dp/1516898672/ref=sr_1_4?ie=UTF8&qid=1460637985&sr=8-4&keywords=brainbuzzz

Maximise your Child's Potential by Sue Cook
http://www.amazon.co.uk/Maximise-your-childs-potential-brainbuzzz/dp/1499246048/ref=sr_1_6?ie=UTF8&qid=1460637985&sr=8-6&keywords=brainbuzzz

Brainbuzzz the Evolution by Sue Cook
http://www.amazon.co.uk/brainbuzzz-evolution-Sue-Cook-ebook/dp/B00B1HHX42/ref=sr_1_1?ie=UTF8&qid=1460637985&sr=8-1&keywords=brainbuzzzSue's websites is www.brainbuzzz.co.uk

Social Media:
YouTube: The Child Brain Whisperer (https://www.youtube.com/channel/UCnhJ8BXUl1pDfxFA7VBGFTQ),

Sue Cook, Brainbuzzz Neuroflow
Look out for brainbuzzz neuroflow, the new brain body exercise class for grown ups who want to retain their healthy brain and body as they age.

Facebook The Child Brain Whisperer (https://www.facebook.com/childbrainwhisperer/?fref=ts) , Brainbuzzz Neuroflow (https://www.facebook.com/Brainbuzzz-Neuroflow-exercise-1128595917183050/?fref=ts) , Brainbuzzz (https://www.facebook.com/Brainbuzzz/?fref=ts) ,

ABOUT THE AUTHOR

Sue Cook is a mum, health scientist, author, trainer, speaker. Before all this, she was a photographer and magazine editor.
Sue likes making things, helping people, and avoiding cooking.
Sue lives in Essex by the sea and fields.

Made in the USA
Charleston, SC
02 July 2016